Fahd

Fahd M. Awwal

Published by Fahd M. Awwal, 2024.

While every precaution has been taken in the preparation of this book, the publisher assumes no responsibility for errors or omissions, or for damages resulting from the use of the information contained herein.

FAHD

First edition. November 2, 2024.

Copyright © 2024 Fahd M. Awwal.

ISBN: 979-8227409874

Written by Fahd M. Awwal.

My humble dedication goes to you, my dear reader, and to all individuals willing to understand the precious power and beauty that resides within every pleasant sleep.

THE POWER AND BEAUTY OF SLEEP

Hi.

It has occurred to me before—the distressing sleep disorder of difficulty falling asleep, staying asleep, and waking up feeling well rested despite having the opportunity for sufficient sleep.

Despite these waking troubles, I feel inspired to share my interesting journey of how I managed to alleviate and overcome this sleep disorder.

Sleep, by nature, is an essential component of our daily lives. However, when each bedtime transforms into a shift from low general vigilance to a sudden plunge into various reflections, we become witnesses to thoughts that our conscience finds unbearable.

For several days over the past few months, I found myself entangled in the restless grip of insomnia. It began subtly, with few nights of tossing and turning, but soon evolved into a nightly struggle against the relentless march of time.

As the world around me surrendered to slumber with the onset of darkness, I would go through my bedtime routine of taking a warm bath and dimming the lights, yet still lie awake, fixedly watching the ticking hands of my bedroom clock as time slipped away. Each second stretched longer, turning my rest into a distant memory. I would stare at the ceiling, the moving fan, or anything I could set my focus on just to pass the stillness in my mind, even watching the midnight shadows dance in the faint moonlight filtering through my curtains.

During those sleepless hours, the world outside took on a surreal quality, as if the veil of normalcy had lifted to reveal a different dimension of life. The usual rhythms of my nightlife felt distorted, with familiar sounds and sights taking on an eerie, almost dreamlike essence.

It was as if I had stepped into an alternate reality where time was suspended, stretching endlessly, and exhaustion was an ever-present companion. Each minute felt like an hour, and each hour like eternity.

Despite the comfort of my bedding, thoughts swirled in my mind like a raging tempest, refusing to grant me the respite I so desperately sought. I could only hang my head and hold my peace.

My days subsequently blurred into a haze of fatigue, where simple tasks transformed into Herculean feats. Even the most mundane activities, like brewing a cup of coffee, required immense effort and concentration. My body felt heavy, and my mind sluggish, challenging my spirit and resolve at every turn. This relentless cycle of wakefulness, coupled with the constant exhaustion of my thoughts, feelings, perception, imagination, remembrance, and will, resembled a never-ending battle against an invisible foe.

It was fanciful to regard this whole encounter as a matter of grave concern because, despite the frustration and weariness, there was a strange beauty in those solitary nights.

In the stillness and silence of the night, I unearthed buried thoughts and emotions, contemplating questions I had long avoided in the busyness of daylight. The darkness became a canvas on which I painted my hopes and fears, seeking solace in the stillness that enveloped me.

I tried everything from herbal teas to meditation, but sleep remained elusive —teasingly close, yet infinitely distant.

Eventually, as mysteriously as it had arrived, my sleep disorder loosened its grip on me. I resorted to both clinical and complementary therapies to treat my sleeplessness, adopting a combination of prescribed medications, cognitive behavioural techniques, mindfulness practices, and natural plant medicine for a more holistic approach.

Consequently, with time and patience, my sleepless nights regained their familiar rhythm, and sleep returned like an old friend, gently pulling me into its comforting embrace. I began to feel waves of relief wash over me with each night as I drifted off more easily, and the dark hours no longer stretched endlessly before me.

Nonetheless, beyond the troubling experience of worry and anxiety lay an indelible mark—a lingering shadow in my consciousness that continually reminded me of the delicate balance between rest and wakefulness. I had come to realize with clarity that sleep is more than just a nightly routine; it is a sanctuary and a refuge where the mind can retreat and rejuvenate.

My sleepless nights, however, were not entirely devoid of revelations. They opened a panoramic window into an alternate reality where time seemed to stand still and thoughts wandered freely in the tranquillity of the night.

I discovered that the mind has its own mysteries to unfold, especially when the world sleeps and the mind wanders alone. Those hours of introspection and solitude brought forth a new understanding of myself and about the world around me, teaching me to cherish the profound silence that accompanies the night and the clarity of thought that often follows a well-rested mind.

The attempt to understand all about sleep is a never-ending journey that begins with the recognition of sleep as not a one-size-fits-all experience.

Sleep is more than just a mere biological function; it ritually calms, graces, and soothes our lives, enriching us in ways we often overlook.

As days transition into nights, sleep calls like a gentle tide, enfolding our body and mind and providing relief from the stress that accumulates with the sun's journey across the sky. This state of surrender welcomes a powerful, quiet, and unseen force that rejuvenates us, stitching together the wear and tear of both mind and muscle. The lingering beauty in this stillness is as elegant as the simple act of closing one's eyes and letting go.

Sleep is the body's sanctuary where restoration occurs without fanfare. During deep sleep, beneath the surface of our consciousness, the body repairs itself by mending the little fractures of daily life. Muscles relax, cells regenerate, and energy replenishes as they await the tasks of tomorrow. In this realm, where dreams begin to flutter at the edge of our awareness, we are at our most vulnerable, yet paradoxically, at our strongest.

It is during these hours of deep sleep that the most profound emotional, physical, and mental healing takes place, ensuring that we awake with renewed strength, ready to face the challenges ahead.

The power of sleep lies in this silent alchemy of renewal and the transformation of exhaustion into vitality.

The restorative power of sleep is not the one and only attribute that renders it essential. The beauty of sleep lies in the tranquillity it offers, providing a peaceful escape where the mind can rest and life's burdens seem to fade away. As Shakespeare wrote, "Sleep that knits up the raveled sleave of care." Sleep serves as a realm where time pauses and the weight of the day dissolves into a soothing stillness. In this serene space, we discover not only physical restoration but also a rare moment of peace for the mind and soul. The descent into sleep resembles falling into a vast ocean of calm, where thoughts drift and dissolve like waves gently breaking on the shore.

The beauty of sleep is delicate and precise, yet profound. It nourishes not just the body but also the spirit, providing a sanctuary where peace and quiet contemplation flourish. It is the silent artist behind life's rhythm, infusing us with grace as it restores us. When morning arrives, the beauty of sleep lingers with a soft glow, carrying us into the day and quietly enriching every waking moment with profound clarity of mind and lightness of heart.

Researchers have identified several sleep disturbances, but we will focus primarily on insomnia, as it is the most common of all sleep disorders.

Insomnia is a sleep disorder that can make it difficult to fall asleep, stay asleep or achieve restful sleep, despite having the opportunity to do so. It often results in daytime impairment and can negatively affect our overall well-being.

Throughout history, insomnia has captivated attention and concern, reflecting the profound impact of sleep on human health, cognition, and quality of life. It is a pervasive disorder that can cast a disruptive shadow over the lives of those affected, hindering their ability to attain adequate and restful sleep. The manifestation of this sleep disturbance varies in intensity and duration, frequently causing significant distress and impairing our daily functioning.

The history of insomnia highlights the enduring quest to understand and address sleep disorders, ensuring that individuals can enjoy restful and rejuvenating nights.

Ancient civilizations throughout Africa and Western Europe acknowledged and documented insomnia as a significant health concern. Ancient medical texts from Egypt, dating back as far as 2000 B.C., not only referenced sleep disorders but also offered detailed descriptions of their symptoms and potential causes. These texts provided remedies and treatment options, including herbal concoctions, meditation techniques, and specific dietary recommendations, all aimed at alleviating the impact of sleeplessness.

The emphasis placed on sleep disorders in these early texts reflect an understanding of the importance of sleep for overall health and well-being.

Philosophers and physicians in ancient times observed sleep disturbances and their effects on human health, recognising that sleeplessness could stem from a range of physical and psychological causes. They noted that lack of sleep could lead to both immediate discomfort and long-term consequences.

These early insights laid the groundwork for understanding insomnia as a multifaceted condition that affects both the body and mind. By acknowledging the complexity of insomnia, they paved the way for future research into its diverse origins and impacts, eventually contributing to the development of more comprehensive treatments and a deeper understanding of sleep disorders in general.

Throughout medieval and Renaissance Europe, there was continual acknowledgement and recognition of insomnia in prominent research and studies. Physicians and scholars during this period explored various theories regarding the causes of sleeplessness, ranging from imbalances of bodily humours to spiritual or psychological disturbances.

The Industrial Revolution and modern era introduced new challenges to sleep patterns. While the rapid pace of industrialization and urbanization intensified concerns about insomnia and its health consequences, the emergence of artificial lighting, shift work, and technological advancements further disrupted the natural sleep-wake cycle for many individuals.

Scientific advancements in the 20th century led to a deeper understanding of sleep physiology and disorders. During this period, experts began to classify insomnia as a clinical condition, defining it by difficulty falling asleep, staying asleep, or waking up too early despite having the opportunity to sleep longer.

Sleeplessness stems from multifaceted causes, including psychological, physiological and environmental factors. Stress and anxiety often trigger a cycle of wakefulness and worry.

Medical conditions like chronic pain, asthma, and gastrointestinal disturbances can also contribute to and intensify insomnia. Additionally, lifestyle choices such as irregular sleep schedules, excessive caffeine intake, and the misuse of electronic devices before bedtime further exacerbate the condition.

Emotional instability frequently follows, leading to increased irritability, mood swings and heightened susceptibility to stress. Physiologically, chronic insomnia raises the risk of cardiovascular disease, obesity, and a weakened immune response.

The complications of insomnia ripple through daily life, impairing cognitive function, mood stability and overall health. Individuals may struggle with concentration, memory, and decision-making.

NATURE OF SLEEP

"I slept like a baby." This common expression typically signifies that you slept soundly and deeply.

Normal human sleep is a state of reduced activity and reactivity, accompanied by low general vigilance. Despite decades of intense scrutiny, our understanding of the natural cause of sleep remains incomplete.

Sleep is a biological process that plays a crucial role in our overall health and well-being, involving a series of stages that the brain cycles through multiple times each night. The transition begins from wakefulness to light sleep during which it is easy for any sound or touch, to wake you. Muscle activity slows down, and occasional muscle twitching may occur. As you move deeper into sleep, your heart rate and breathing slow, and body temperature drops.

While there is a decreased ability to react to environmental stimuli during sleep, this does not imply that the body and brain are on vacation. Instead, the brain remains highly active throughout the night, facilitating many essential functions beneath our consciousness.

There is something incredibly peaceful about the act of sleeping itself. It is a time when the world fades away and we transition to a state of rest and rejuvenation. The quiet and stillness of sleep provide a much-needed break from the hustle and bustle of daily life.

Overall, the driving force of sleep lies in its ability to nurture and renew us, helping us face each day with a refreshed perspective and outlook.

KEY QUALITIES OF GOOD SLEEP

As the evening settles and the world quiets down, the promise of good sleep beckons. Good sleep is not just about the hours spent in bed, but the kind of rest that truly restores you. It is like slipping into a gentle rhythm where both your body and mind find their way to peace.

The key to good sleep starts with consistency. Imagine lying down at the same time each night to help your body become familiar with this bedtime routine. Your mind learns that it is time to rest, and soon, you will find yourself slipping into slumber without much effort. The minutes will not stretch on endlessly as you lie awake but instead, you will be on the edge of a dream within 10 or 20 minutes.

Once you are there, deep in the night, there is nothing but uninterrupted calm. You will not wake every hour, and even if you do, it will be brief with your body rolling back into that comforting heaviness as you fall asleep again easily. There is no tossing and turning, no battling with pillows or sheets. Everything is peaceful. The room is dark, quiet, and the air is just cool enough to invite deeper sleep.

Meanwhile, in the background, your organs are at work. The moment is not just about sleep; it is also about restoration. Your muscles, tired from the day, are rebuilding. Your mind, perhaps weighed down with worries or stress, is sorting through thoughts in the dream world, healing and organizing. Deep sleep cradles you like a sanctuary as the silent power of the night knits together everything that needs repair.

Then morning comes, not with a jolt, but with ease. You wake up feeling relieved, clear-headed, and energised, as though the night has given you exactly what you need. Your mind feels alert, your emotions steady. The irritability, fatigue, and stress are gone and replaced by a kind of calm readiness. This is the true gift of good sleep.

Throughout the day, the benefits of that night's sleep linger. You do not find yourself yearning for a nap or feeling the weight of exhaustion pulling at your eyes. Instead, there is focus, creativity, and an energy that sustains you —all thanks to the simple yet powerful act of sleeping well.

Sleep Cycles

When thinking about getting the sleep you need, it is common to focus on how many hours of sleep you will get. While sleep duration is undoubtedly important, it is just a fraction of the entire sleep equation.

The sleep cycle is a repeating pattern of stages that our brain and body go through during sleep. This process is dynamic and non-static, with each stage contributing uniquely to restorative sleep and overall well-being. A complete sleep cycle lasts about 90 minutes, with the body alternating between Non-Rapid Eye Movement (NREM) and Rapid Eye Movement (REM) stages. A typical night includes four to six cycles, with Non-Rapid Eye Movement Sleep dominating the early part of the night and Rapid Eye Movement Sleep becoming more prominent toward morning.

Each sleep stage plays a vital role in different aspects of health, highlighting that the quality and composition of sleep are just as important as the total hours of sleep. To achieve restful and restorative sleep, it is essential to ensure the right balance of all sleep stages throughout the night.

Stage 1: Non-Rapid Eye Movement Sleep

This is the lightest stage of sleep that marks the transition from wakefulness to slumber. It is easy to wake someone in this state because the body and mind have just begun to relax. Sleepers may experience brief muscle twitches or a sensation of falling, often accompanied by fleeting thoughts and random dream-like sensations. This stage is very short, lasting only a few minutes, and serves as the gateway to deeper sleep stages. While brain activity starts to slow down, it remains moderately active, making this stage less restful than the subsequent ones.

Stage 2: Non-Rapid Eye Movement Sleep

This stage represents a deeper and more stable phase of sleep during which the body's systems begin to slow down in preparation for even deeper sleep. During this stage, body temperature drops, heart rate slows, and muscles relax further. Brain activity decreases significantly compared to Stage 1, but occasional bursts of rapid brain waves, known as sleep spindles and K-complexes, characterize this stage. Experts believe that these brain activities play a role in memory consolidation and sensory processing. This stage of sleep is vital for maintaining overall sleep quality and usually lasts about 20 minutes during the first sleep cycle, progressively becoming longer with each subsequent cycle.

Stage 3: Non-Rapid Eye Movement Sleep

Also known as deep sleep or slow-wave sleep (SWS). This is the most restorative sleep stage. It is crucial for physical restoration, tissue repair, and immune function, as well as for the release of growth hormones. During this stage, brain waves are at their slowest, making it very difficult to awaken someone. If roused during this stage, a person is likely to feel disoriented or groggy. Stage 3 is essential for waking up feeling refreshed and rejuvenated, but it becomes shorter as the night progresses, allowing for more time in Rapid Eye Movement (REM) sleep.

Stage 4: Rapid Eye Movement Sleep

Rapid Eye Movement (REM) sleep is characterised by rapid eye movements, vivid dreaming, and increased brain activity. REM sleep is essential for memory consolidation, learning, and emotional regulation. As the night progresses, the periods of REM sleep lengthen, with the longest phase occurring in the early morning hours.

Most dreams occur during Rapid Eye Movement (REM) sleep, which get its name from the rapid movement of the eyes behind the eyelids while dreaming. During REM sleep, brain activity closely resembles that of being awake, indicating that the brain is highly active, processing information and preparing for wakefulness.

Understanding sleep cycles can help you optimize your sleep. For example, waking up during a deep sleep phase can leave you feeling groggy, while waking up at the end of a cycle can make you feel more refreshed. This is why sleep experts often recommend trying to wake up at the end of a complete cycle. Tools like sleep trackers and apps can be helpful for setting optimal wake-up times.

Maintaining a consistent sleep schedule, such as going to bed and waking up at the same time each day, along with creating a sleep-friendly environment that has optimal room temperature and is free from distractions, is essential for organising good sleep architecture. These techniques help support and preserve healthy sleep, ensuring that our bodies and minds receive the necessary restorative benefits throughout the night.

BASIC FUNCTIONS OF SLEEP

In the stillness of the night, as the world settles into a gentle hush, your body embarks on a journey into a realm of restoration. The soft embrace of your bed welcomes you, the weight of the day gradually lifting as you sink into comfort. As your eyes close, the first threads of sleep weave together, pulling you deeper into a state of calm.

The initial lightness of slumber washes over you as a prelude to the deeper rest that awaits. Your breathing slows, becoming steady and rhythmic as your heart rate follows suit, settling into a tranquil beat. This marks the beginning of your body's nightly ritual, where every cell, muscle, and tissue starts to repair and rejuvenate.

As you drift further into sleep, your body enters the deep and restorative stages. In the quiet depths of your slumber, your muscles relax completely, free from the tension and strain of the day. Released growth hormone works tirelessly to mend the microtears in your muscles, strengthening them for the challenges of tomorrow. Your ever-vigilant immune system uses this time to bolster its defences by producing the proteins and antibodies that will protect you from illnesses.

Initially, the transition into sleep is gentle, like the soft lull of a lullaby. Your breathing slows, your heart rate eases and your body gradually releases its grip on the day's stress. As you enter this calm state, the first hints of sleep's many functions begin to reveal themselves.

Sleep for RESTORATION

Sleep is a powerful force of restoration, serving essential processes that enable the body to repair, heal, rejuvenate, and prepare for the demands of the day ahead. When you sleep, especially during the deep sleep stages, your body enters a state of intense repair and recovery. This is when your muscles, bones, and tissues undergo crucial maintenance.

Imagine your body as a finely tuned machine that has been working hard all day. During sleep, this machine receives the care it needs: the worn-out parts get repaired, the energy reserves become replenished, and any damage is fixed. This is particularly important for those who are physically active, as muscles recover and grow stronger during these hours of rest.

The release of growth hormones during deep sleep is a key aspect of this restoration process. These hormones play a vital role in repairing tissues, building muscle, and even supporting healthy metabolism. They ensure that your body is not just resting but also growing, strengthening, and laying down new tissues, so you wake up feeling physically revitalized.

The restoration does not stop at the muscles and tissues. Sleep also plays a crucial role in detoxifying your body. During sleep, your brain initiates the removal of toxins that accumulate throughout the day. This cleansing process is essential for maintaining healthy brain function and preventing cognitive decline. It is as if your body is running a deep-cleaning program, clearing out waste and harmful substances so that every system operates smoothly.

On a cellular level, sleep is a time for renewal. Cells throughout your body regenerate, replacing old and damaged cells with new and healthy ones. This continuous cycle of cell turnover is vital for maintaining everything from your skin's health and appearance to the proper functioning of your organs.

Athletes and physically active individuals gain significant benefits from restorative sleep, as it enhances physical performance, speed, agility, and endurance. A good night's sleep leads to a more positive mood, increased energy, and an improved overall quality of life.

Sleep serves as your body's ultimate restoration tool. It is a time when every system in the body receives the care and attention it needs to function optimally. Without sufficient sleep, your body struggles to repair itself, resulting in fatigue, weakened immunity, and a general sense of feeling down. With quality sleep, you awaken feeling refreshed, strong, and ready to tackle whatever the day brings, knowing that your body has undergone deep restorative sleep.

Sleep for COGNITIVE FUNCTION and MEMORY CONSOLIDATION

Sleep plays a crucial role in cognitive function and memory consolidation by acting as a vital process that strengthens your mind and enhances learning.

Throughout the day, your brain continually absorbs information—everything from facts to experiences and emotions. This influx of information can be overwhelming, akin to sorting through a cluttered desk filled with papers, notes, and reminders. When you sleep, your brain takes on the role of an efficient organizer, carefully sifting through all that information.

As you enter the deeper stages of sleep, particularly Rapid Eye Movement (REM) sleep, your brain becomes highly active. This is when memory consolidation occurs. Your brain sorts through the day's experiences and decides what to retain and what to discard. It is like a librarian, meticulously cataloguing books and ensuring that knowledge is preserved and readily accessible.

This process is essential for learning, problem-solving, and overall mental acuity. It involves strengthening and storing important memories, such as studying for an exam or acquiring a new skill for future use, while also pruning away less critical information. This is similar to cataloguing and filing books, ensuring that everything is in its proper place and easy to find when needed.

Without adequate sleep, your brain struggles to retain and integrate new information with what you already know. It is like trying to build a puzzle with missing pieces; everything feels disjointed and incomplete. However, with sufficient sleep, those pieces come together to create a clear and cohesive picture.

Deep sleep enhances cognitive function by clearing out toxins that accumulate in the brain during the day. This cleansing process keeps your mind fresh, just like resetting a computer to improve its performance. It allows you to wake up with a clear head, ready to tackle new challenges, solve problems, and think creatively while maintaining mental sharpness and focus.

In essence, sleep is your brain's way of ensuring that the knowledge you acquire is not only retained but also accessible and usable. During these quiet hours, your mind performs its most important work of organizing and solidifying memories, sharpening cognitive abilities, and preparing you to learn and grow each day.

Sleep for EMOTIONAL REGULATION

Sleep has a profound connection with emotional regulation, serving as a stabilizer for our mood and emotional well-being. When we sleep, the brain engages in a complex process that aids in processing emotions, managing stress, and maintaining a balanced emotional state.

Throughout the day, we encounter a wide range of emotions, including joy, frustration, excitement, and anxiety. These emotions can be intense and overwhelming, leaving the brain with so much to process. During sleep, particularly in the Rapid Eye Movement (REM) sleep stage, the brain seizes the opportunity to sort through these emotions. It is as if the brain is performing a nightly "emotional reset", processing and making sense of the day's experiences.

During REM sleep, the brain replays emotional experiences and integrates them with existing memories. This helps desensitize emotional responses, taking the edge off intense feelings. For instance, if something upsetting occurs during the day, REM sleep can help soften the emotional impact, allowing you to wake up feeling more at peace with the situation.

It is like a therapist working through your feelings, helping you understand and manage them in a healthier way.

This process also involves the brain's stress response system. Sleep helps regulate cortisol, the stress hormone, ensuring that it remains at appropriate levels. Without adequate sleep, cortisol levels can stay elevated, leading to increased feelings of stress and anxiety. Over time, this can make it harder to cope with everyday challenges, as your emotional resilience begins to erode.

Moreover, sleep helps to balance the amygdala, the part of the brain that controls emotions, particularly fear and anger. When you are sleep-deprived, the amygdala becomes more reactive, thus leading to heightened emotional responses. This can make you more susceptible to irritability, mood swings, and impulsive reactions. With adequate sleep, reactions to emotional stimuli become more measured and rational, aiding in regulating the amygdala.

In addition to managing stress and balancing emotions, sleep plays a key role in empathy and social interactions. During sleep, the brain processes social cues and emotional nuances, helping you better understand and connect with others. This emotional insight is essential for healthy relationships, as it enables you to respond to others with sensitivity and compassion.

In essence, sleep is your brain's way of maintaining balance in your emotional world. It helps you process life's difficulties by ensuring that you wake up with a clearer and calmer perspective. When sleep is disrupted, emotional regulation suffers, leading to increased stress, anxiety and emotional instability. However, with sufficient sleep, you are better equipped to handle whatever comes your way, thus maintaining emotional equilibrium and a more positive outlook to life.

Sleep for
IMMUNE SYSTEM SUPPORT

Sleep is an essential ally of the immune system, serving as a period when the body strengthens its defences against illness and infection.

During sleep, especially in the deeper stages, the body engages in essential processes that enhance immune function, helping to keep you healthy and resilient.

Throughout the day, your body encounter various pathogens such as bacteria, viruses, and other invaders that can jeopardise your health. Your immune system continuously works identify and neutralize these threats. However, this defence system needs rest and recovery to function optimally, and this is where sleep comes in.

During deep sleep, the body boosts the production of cytokines. These small proteins are crucial in controlling the growth and activity of other immune system cells and blood cells. When released, they signal the immune system to do its job. Theses cytokines have a protective effect that aids in the fight against infections and reduces inflammation. They act as messengers, signalling the immune system to increase its activity upon detecting a threat. Without sufficient sleep, there is a decrease in the production of these essential cytokines, and this in turn weakens the body's ability to respond to infections.

Sleep also supports the immune system by promoting the production of T-cells, a type of white blood cell. T-cells are crucial for recognizing and attacking infected cells, playing a significant role in the body's defence against illness. During sleep, T-cells become more effective at their function, as there is an increase in their ability to adhere to and destroy infected cells. This process ensures that your immune system is always prepared to respond quickly and effectively to any invaders.

In addition to boosting cytokine and T-cell production, sleep plays a crucial role in regulating other immune functions. For instance, it aids the production of antibodies, which are proteins that specifically target and neutralize pathogens. Antibodies act as the body's custom-made weapons, designed to recognize and eliminate specific invaders. With adequate sleep, the body can produce these antibodies more efficiently, thus offering stronger protection against diseases.

Furthermore, sleep is a time when the body repairs and regenerates its cells including those of the immune system. This renewal process ensures that your immune cells remain healthy and function optimally to shield you from illness. Any disruption or deficiency in sleep diminishes the immune system's ability to defend the body. This occurs due to a compromise in the body's repair processes, leaving the immune system less capable of providing adequate protection.

Sleep also helps regulate inflammation, which is a natural response to infection or injury. Inflammation occurs when the body releases chemicals that trigger an immune response to fight off infection or heal damaged tissue. Once the body heals the injury or infection, the inflammation process ends. While inflammation is essential for healing, chronic inflammation can lead to various health issues including weakened immune function. During deep sleep, the body works to balance inflammation in ways that support recovery without causing harm.

Without sufficient sleep, the immune system becomes less effective, thus increasing the risk of illnesses and prolonging recovery times. With adequate sleep, your body is better equipped to fend off infections and heal more quickly to maintain a good balance between your health and immunity.

Sleep for PSYCHOLOGICAL and MENTAL WELLBEING

Sleep is the cornerstone of psychological and mental wellbeing. It provides your brain with the necessary time to rest and maintain emotional balance. When we sleep, the mind undergoes several crucial processes that support mental well-being, resilience and overall psychological stability.

Throughout the day, the brain is constantly processing information, making decisions and navigating stress. This mental activity takes a toll that leads to the accumulation of cognitive and emotional fatigue. Sleep acts as a powerful antidote to this wear and tear, allowing the brain to reset and recharge, restoring its ability to function optimally

When there is a disruption or insufficiency in sleep, cognitive processes become impaired, resulting in difficulties with attention, memory, and executive functioning. Over time, chronic sleep deprivation can contribute to mental health issues such as depression and anxiety, as the brain struggles to cope with the demands of daily life.

Furthermore, sleep is essential for maintaining a positive outlook and emotional resilience. Sleep-deprived individuals are more likely to experience negative moods, irritability and pessimism. This is partly because sleep deprivation affects the brain's ability to regulate emotions, leading to increased sensitivity to stress and negative stimuli. Conversely, good-quality sleep enhances emotional stability by helping you to cope with challenges, maintain a positive outlook and interact with others more effectively.

Deep sleep is crucial for preventing and managing mental health disorders. Sleep disturbances closely link to conditions like depression, anxiety, and bipolar disorder. Poor sleep hygiene can exacerbate symptoms of these conditions by creating a vicious cycle where mental health issues lead to sleep problems, which in turn worsen mental health. On the other hand, improving sleep quality can be a key component of treatment for these disorders, helping to stabilize mood, reduce symptoms, and improve overall well-being.

Sleep for METABOLIC AND CARDIOVASCULAR HEALTH

Sleep is a vital force that sustains the intricate balance of your metabolic and cardiovascular health. As you drift into slumber, your body does not simply rest; it engages in a series of processes that help regulate metabolism, support heart health, and reduce the risk of chronic diseases.

One of the primary ways sleep influences metabolic health is through its impact on hormone regulation. During sleep, the body balances the levels of key hormones that control hunger and appetite such as leptin and ghrelin. Leptin signals fullness while ghrelin stimulates hunger. When you don't get enough sleep, leptin levels decrease and ghrelin levels increase, leading to heightened appetite and cravings, particularly for high-calorie, carbohydrate-rich foods. This hormonal imbalance can result in overeating and weight gain, thereby increasing the risk of obesity.

Sleep also affects insulin sensitivity, which is crucial for maintaining healthy blood sugar levels. Insulin is the hormone that allows cells to absorb glucose from the bloodstream and use it for energy. When you are sleep-deprived, your body becomes less sensitive to insulin, necessitating the production of more of the hormone to achieve the same effect. This condition, known as insulin resistance, is a significant risk factor for developing type 2 diabetes. Consistently poor sleep can lead to chronically elevated blood sugar levels, further increasing the risk of metabolic disorders.

Beyond metabolism, sleep plays an essential role in cardiovascular health. In the depths of deep sleep, the body experiences a natural drop in heart rate and blood pressure, providing the cardiovascular system with much-needed rest. This nightly dip allows the heart to recover from the demands of the day, easing strain on the heart and blood vessels. Over time, this restorative process fosters healthy blood pressure levels and lowers the risk of hypertension—a leading cause of heart disease and stroke.

Sleep also plays a role in regulating inflammation, which has a close connection to cardiovascular health. Chronic inflammation significantly contributes to the development of atherosclerosis—the build-up of plaque in the arteries, which can precipitate heart attacks and strokes. During sleep, the body curtails the production of pro-inflammatory molecules, helping to keep inflammation in check and protecting the cardiovascular system from damage.

Furthermore, sleep deprivation is associated with an increased risk of developing arrhythmias (irregular heartbeats), heart failure, and coronary artery disease. Insufficient sleep elevates stress hormones like cortisol, which can place additional strain on the heart. Over time, this heightened stress can weaken the cardiovascular system, making it more vulnerable to conditions such as diseased vessels, structural problems, and blood clots.

Deep sleep also helps regulate cholesterol levels. Adequate sleep supports the production of High-Density Lipoprotein (HDL), often referred to as "good" cholesterol, which helps remove Low-Density Lipoprotein (LDL) or "bad" cholesterol from the arteries. This balance is essential in preventing plaque accumulation in the arteries that can lead to heart disease.

In essence, sleep nurtures our metabolic functions and supports our cardiovascular system, reminding us that restful nights are foundational to a vibrant and healthy life.

CULTURE OF SLEEP

The culture of sleep is an intricate and fascinating tapestry woven from various traditions, beliefs and practices that shape how different societies approach rest and relaxation. Sleep is not merely a biological necessity but also a cultural phenomenon, reflecting a wide array of values, customs and societal norms across the globe.

Many indigenous cultures perceive sleep as a state of divinity, during which the mind and body are renewed and restored. For instance, in Japanese culture, the concept of "inemuri" allows people to sleep in public workplaces or on public transport without stigma. This practice indicates dedication and hard work, suggesting that individuals can fall asleep wherever they find themselves.

The concept of "inemuri" embodies a cultural understanding that sleep is not just a private matter but also an integral part of daily life, reflecting one's commitment to work and community.

In contrast, many Western cultures emphasize the importance of uninterrupted, private sleep. There is a strong emphasis on the need for a full eight hours of sleep in a quiet, dark room as essential for health and productivity. This focus on sleep as a private, personal experience mirrors a broader societal value placed on individual health and well-being. The rise of sleep science and wellness culture in these societies has led to a proliferation of sleep aids like high-tech mattresses and sleep-tracking devices. These practices underscore the importance placed on optimizing sleep quality.

Various cultures also exhibit diverse practices regarding sleep environments and rituals. In some Middle Eastern and Latin American cultures, communal sleeping arrangements are prevalent. Families may sleep together in a single room or even a single bed. This practice reflects close-knit family bonding and the cultural values woven around togetherness and support. Such communal sleeping practices can foster a strong sense of security and connection among family members.

In many cultures, sleep rituals and bedtime routines serve as opportunities for storytelling and social bonding. In western cultures, for instance, bedtime stories are cherished traditions that aim to nurture children's imagination and strengthen parent-child relationships. Moreover, some Indigenous cultures incorporate sleep into their broader spiritual practices, viewing dreams as messages from ancestors or the spirit world. These cultures may have specific rituals or practices designed to encourage meaningful dreaming or to honour the insights gained from dreams.

The concept of siesta—a short nap taken in the early afternoon, is another cultural practice related to sleep. In Mediterranean and Latin American countries like Spain and Mexico, the siesta is a traditional part of daily life, reflecting the cultural value placed on rest and relaxation during the day. This practice is often integral to work schedules and daily routines, highlighting a cultural attitude that prioritizes well-being over continuous productivity.

Conversely, the widespread use of smartphones and electronic devices has introduced new challenges and alterations to sleep patterns on a global trend. Many cultures now contend with the effects of "digital insomnia", where screen usage before bedtime disrupts sleep. This has led to a growing cultural focus on "sleep hygiene", a phenomenon that promotes the good value of healthy sleep practices, such as reducing screen time before bed and establishing calming bedtime routines.

The amount of sleep a person needs as well as their preference for waking early or staying up late, varies from individual to individual. Understanding the cultural context of sleep can provide valuable insights into how different societies prioritize and approach rest, ultimately influencing individual sleep behaviours and public health initiatives.

The culture of sleep is a rich and diverse field that reflects a myriad of traditions, values, and practices varying across different societies.

From communal sleeping arrangements to individual sleep optimization, cultural attitudes toward sleep reveal much about how societies prioritize rest, health and well-being. Sleep is not only a biological necessity but also a cultural artefact shaped by, and shaping the ways we live and interact with one another.

Here are some aspects of how various cultures approach rest and sleep:

SIESTAS AND NAPPING

In many cultures around the world, people weave the concepts of siestas and napping into the fabric of daily life. They embody a unique approach to sleep that values rest and rejuvenation as integral parts of the daily routine.

The siesta, a traditional midday nap, is a cultural hallmark in several Mediterranean and Latin American countries. In Spain, for instance, the siesta is a beloved tradition that reflects the country's emphasis on balancing work and enjoyment of life. Traditionally, the siesta occurs after lunch, often between 2pm and 4pm, when the sun is at its peak and temperatures soar. This pause in the day provides a much-needed respite from the heat, allowing people to recharge before continuing with their daily activities. In Spanish culture, the siesta is a time to unwind, relax and rejuvenate, often accompanied by a light meal or a social gathering. This practice not only supports physical well-being but also fosters a sense of community and connection.

Similarly, in Mexico and other Latin American countries, the tradition of the siesta is an essential part of daily life. It is a time when businesses may pause and families gather to rest and enjoy each other's company. The siesta is a cherished part of their cultural rhythm, offering a moment of respite amid a busy day. It reflects a cultural value that emphasises balance of work and quality of life, acknowledging that rest is as vital as productivity.

In Italy, the concept of "riposo" serves a similar purpose. Italians often take a break after lunch to relax and recharge. This practice underscores the cultural appreciation for both food and rest. This period of rest is viewed as a means to maintain energy levels and ensure a more enjoyable and productive afternoon.

In other parts of Asia, such as China and Korea, short naps are commonly accepted and encouraged. These brief periods of rest, often referred to as "power naps," are essential to the workday for boosting productivity and focus. This approach reflects a cultural understanding that sleep and rest are vital for maintaining mental sharpness and overall well-being.

The growing recognition of the benefits of napping and midday rest is also evident in modern global wellness trends. Many health experts advocate for short naps as a means to enhance cognitive function, improve mood and increase productivity. This aligns with traditional practices of siestas and napping, reinforcing the idea that rest is a crucial component of a healthy and balanced lifestyle.

Siestas and napping symbolize a cultural celebration of rest and rejuvenation. These practices have deep roots in various traditions and reflect a broader cultural value that emphasizes the significance of work-life balance. By finding the right balance, individuals can improve their physical and mental health, increase productivity, reduce stress, and cultivate stronger relationships. Whether it is the beloved midday nap in Spain, the riposo in Italy, or public napping in Japan, these cultural approaches to sleep underscore a shared understanding that rest is not only a personal necessity but also a cultural practice that enhances quality of life and fosters community and social bonding.

POLYPHASIC SLEEP PATTERNS

Polyphasic sleep patterns involve breaking sleep into multiple segments throughout the day rather than a single consolidated period. This concept presents a fascinating and varied approach to rest that reflects different cultural and historical attitudes towards sleep.

Historically, polyphasic sleep was a common practice before the advent of electric lighting. In many pre-industrial societies, people followed a natural rhythm that included two main sleep periods: the first sleep and the second sleep. This biphasic sleep pattern was marked by a period of rest during the night, followed by a wakeful period in the early hours, and then a return to sleep until morning. During this wakeful period, people might engage in quiet activities such as reading, praying or socialising. The natural light-to-darkness cycle and the needs of pre-modern life significantly influenced this sleep pattern, often requiring people to adapt their sleep patterns to their environment and activities.

In contemporary times, polyphasic sleep has seen a revival as some individuals explore it as an alternative to the traditional monophasic sleep schedule, which involves a single uninterrupted period of sleep at night. Advocates of polyphasic sleep argue that dividing sleep into multiple periods can lead to increased productivity through more efficient use of time. This concept has gained attention in various cultures and subcultures, reflecting a diverse range of attitudes toward sleep.

One well-known polyphasic sleep pattern is the Uberman sleep schedule, which involves taking short 20-minute naps every four hours throughout the day. Advocates of this schedule believe it maximizes waking hours and enhances cognitive performance by prioritizing Rapid Eye Movement (REM) sleep, which is particularly restorative. This schedule embodies a modern, efficiency-oriented approach to sleep by emphasizing the desire to optimize productivity and wakefulness.

Another example is the Everyman sleep schedule, which combines a core sleep period with several short naps throughout the day. This approach allows for a longer block of sleep at night, supplemented by additional naps to maintain alertness and reduce overall sleep time. This pattern reflects a more balanced approach to polyphasic sleep, integrating longer sleep periods with strategic napping to manage sleep needs and daily responsibilities.

In highly stressed environments or professions with irregular hours, such as healthcare or the military, individuals may embrace polyphasic sleep to accommodate unconventional work schedules and ensure they remain functional and alert. In these contexts, polyphasic sleep becomes a practical adaptation to the demands of modern life, reflecting a broader cultural shift toward flexibility and adaptability in sleep practices.

These sleep patterns demonstrate how attitudes towards sleep continue to adapt and transform. They underscore the ongoing quest to balance rest with productivity, optimize health and align sleep with the demands and opportunities of modern life.

BED SHARING AND CO-SLEEPING

Bed sharing and co-sleeping are practices deeply rooted in cultural traditions, family dynamics and historical customs. They reflect a diverse array of values and beliefs about rest, family bonding and the nurturing of children.

Bed Sharing

Bed sharing, or the practice of sleeping in the same bed with one or more family members, is a well-known tradition among several cultures in many parts of the world. It symbolizes close bonding and collective well-being, making it an integral part of daily life.

In many Asian cultures, such as Japan and China, it is customary for families to sleep together in a shared space. In Japan, people often spread out traditional futons on the floor of a shared room, allowing family members to sleep close to one another. This practice is rooted in values of family cohesion and support, wherein close physical proximity fosters emotional security and maintains strong family connections.

In parts of Latin America, families often sleep together in a single bed or room, reflecting cultural values of unity and mutual support. This practice nurtures children by providing them with a sense of security and comfort during their formative years.

Co-Sleeping

Co-sleeping, which involves sharing a sleep space with infants or young children, is another culturally significant practice. It often entails having a child sleep in the same bed or room as their parents. This practice varies widely across cultures, with different communities holding distinct attitudes and traditions regarding it.

Many traditional cultures view co-sleeping as a practical way to promote family bonding and ensure that children receive close physical and emotional support. Parents believe that sleeping near their children strengthens the parent-child relationship and fosters a sense of safety and security.

In contrast, Western cultures have traditionally favoured separate sleeping arrangements for infants and parents, emphasizing independence and safe sleep practices. However, recent shifts in cultural attitudes have sparked renewed interest in co-sleeping, with some parents adopting the practice for its perceived benefits in bonding and night care.

Bed sharing and co-sleeping reflect deeper cultural values and beliefs about family life and child rearing. In cultures where these practices are common, they often signify a strong emphasis on family togetherness, emotional security, and mutual support. The close physical proximity of bed sharing and co-sleeping enhances emotional connections, provides comfort, and fosters a nurturing environment for children.

In cultures where separate sleeping arrangements are more prevalent, there is often a focus on encouraging independence and establishing boundaries. This approach may reflect values of self-reliance and personal space, emphasizing the importance of individual sleep needs as well as the benefits of a separate sleep environment.

In contemporary times, the practice of bed sharing and co-sleeping influence cultural traditions and modern research. Some studies highlight the potential benefits of co-sleeping, such as easier night breastfeeding and improved infant sleep patterns. At the same time, concerns about safety and sleep quality have led to recommendations for safe sleep practices, including the use of separate sleep surfaces for infants.

CULTURAL ATTITUDES TOWARD SLEEP DURATION

Cultural attitudes toward sleep duration reveal a fascinating spectrum of beliefs and practices that reflect varying values about health, productivity, and daily life. These attitudes shape how societies perceive the amount of sleep deemed optimal and acceptable, thereby influencing both individual habits and broader societal norms.

In many **Western cultures**, the standard for sleep duration often revolves around the recommendation of approximately 7-9 hours per night for adults. Research supports this benchmark by linking adequate sleep with improved health outcomes, cognitive function, and emotional well-being. In these cultures, there is a significant emphasis on the concept of "good sleep hygiene," which includes maintaining consistent sleep schedules, creating restful environments and minimizing disruptions.

However, prevailing cultural narratives equate longer hours of wakefulness with productivity and success. The "hustle culture," prevalent in many Western societies, often glorifies the ability to function on minimal sleep as a benchmark of ambition and drive.

This attitude can lead to sleep deprivation and a disregard for the importance of rest, as individuals may prioritize work and other obligations over their sleep needs.

In **Mediterranean and Latin American cultures**, the concept of midday rest or the siesta reflects a different approach to sleep duration. In these regions, people often divide the day into two segments: a period of work, followed by a midday break for rest or a nap and then a continuation of work in the late afternoon. This cultural attitude values balance and recuperation, with the siesta serving as an important part of daily life that acknowledges the natural need for rest and helps mitigate the effects of the afternoon slump.

This approach contrasts with the more continuous workday model seen in some other cultures, thereby highlighting how regional practices can shape attitudes toward sleep duration and daily life.

In various **Indigenous and traditional cultures**, people often closely align sleep duration with natural rhythms and the demands of daily life.

For example, in many Indigenous communities, sleep patterns are more flexible and synchronized with natural light cycles and seasonal changes. Rest and sleep are integral parts of daily routines, reflecting a deep connection with the environment and a holistic understanding of well-being.

These cultures often view sleep as a natural and essential part of life, placing less emphasis on strict sleep duration guidelines and more focus on the quality and alignment of rest with natural rhythms.

In the **modern global context**, scientific research and health trends increasingly influence attitudes toward sleep duration. There is a growing awareness of the importance of sufficient sleep for overall health and well-being, with many health organizations advocating for the 7-9 hours of sleep recommendation. Additionally, the rise of wellness and self-care movements has led to increased attention to sleep quality and the impact of lifestyle factors on sleep duration.

At the same time, the global nature of modern work and technology has introduced new challenges, such as the effects of screen time and irregular working hours on sleep patterns. This has led to an increased focus on sleep management strategies and the importance of balancing sleep with other aspects of a busy and connected lifestyle.

SLEEP AND SOCIAL STATUS

There is an intricate connection between sleep and social status, with cultural norms and societal structures often influencing and reflecting how different groups perceive and experience rest. This relationship highlights how sleep is not merely a personal necessity but also a strong indicator of social status and class.

Historically, the relationship between sleep and social status has been evident in the lifestyles of different social classes. In pre-industrial societies, people largely dictate sleep patterns by the availability of resources and societal roles. Nobility and wealthy classes often enjoyed the luxury of extended sleep and rest, with private sleeping quarters and comfortable bedding. In contrast, lower social classes, including labourers and peasants, typically had more irregular sleep patterns, often due to the demands of manual labour and limited access to comfortable sleeping arrangements.

The differentiation in sleep quality and duration between social classes was not just a matter of comfort but also of societal value. Those with higher social status could afford to prioritize rest and recuperation while those of lower status often had to sacrifice sleep for economic survival.

In contemporary society, the connection between sleep and social status continues to manifest in various ways. Access to quality sleep is often associated with socioeconomic factors, including income, education, and employment. Individuals with higher incomes and educational levels are more likely to have access to environments conducive to good sleep, such as private bedrooms, high-quality mattresses, and controlled temperature conditions. They also tend to have the flexibility to prioritize sleep, taking advantage of opportunities for rest and relaxation.

In contrast, those with lower incomes or demanding low-wage jobs may encounter more challenges in achieving quality sleep. Irregular work hours, multiple jobs, and high levels of stress can disrupt sleep patterns, ultimately leading to shorter sleep duration and poorer sleep quality.

Additionally, living conditions such as noisy environments, overcrowded housing, and limited access to healthcare can further affect sleep. This disparity in sleep access and quality reflects broader social inequalities, where sleep becomes an indicator of privilege and resources.

In some cultures, the ability to sleep well symbolises success and high social standing. For example, in many Western societies, the emphasis on achieving a full eight hours of sleep is often associated with self-care and personal well-being, which are viewed as indicators of a balanced and successful life. Those who can prioritize sleep and manage their health effectively are often more affluent and in control of their lives.

Conversely, in high-pressure environments, such as competitive corporate or academic settings, long working hours and sleep deprivation are symbols of dedication and ambition. In these contexts, individuals may see sacrificing sleep for work or achievement as a badge of honour that reflects their commitment to career success and social advancement.

The relationship between **sleep and professional success** further illustrates the connection between sleep and social status. High-status professions often provide greater flexibility and working conditions that support regular sleep patterns. Executives, academics, and professionals in certain fields may have more control over their schedules, enabling them to prioritize rest and maintain healthy sleep habits.

In contrast, lower-status jobs, particularly those involving shift work, long hours, or physically demanding tasks, can disrupt regular sleep. This not only affects sleep quality but can also have implications for overall health and career advancement. The impact of sleep on job performance and health underscores the broader societal implications of sleep and social status.

SLEEP ENVIRONMENT AND PRACTICES

Sleep environments and practices have deep roots in cultural contexts, reflecting diverse values, traditions and beliefs about rest and well-being. These cultural attitudes shape the design and structure of sleep spaces and routines, as well as society's perception of the importance of sleep.

In many **traditional cultures**, the design and use of sleep environments have a strong correlation with communal living and cultural practices. For instance, in numerous Asian cultures, traditional sleeping arrangements often involve resting on the floor using futons or mats.

In Japan, the use of "tatami" mats alongside "futons" exemplifies a practical and space-efficient approach to sleep, where rolling and storing them during the day aligns with cultural values of simplicity and multifunctional use of space.

In some **Indigenous cultures**, people harmoniously design sleep environments in relation to the natural world. For example, many Native American tribes historically utilized sleeping arrangements that mirrored their nomadic lifestyles, such as sleeping on animal hides or woven mats. These setups were crafted to provide comfort while also being easily transportable, reflecting a profound connection to the environment and a practical approach to living.

In **contemporary societies**, the sleep environment has become more specialized and individualized, influenced by modern comforts and technological advancements. High-quality mattresses, adjustable beds, and temperature control systems are now prevalent in many Western households.

This reflects the cultural emphasis on optimizing sleep for health and comfort. The focus on creating an ideal sleep environment includes considerations such as lighting, noise reduction, and temperature control, as well as the use of high-thread-count bedsheets and maintaining a consistent sleep schedule—all aimed at enhancing the quality of rest.

In **lower-income** settings or regions with limited resources, sleep environments may be more modest and less specialized. Sleep practices in these contexts may reflect practical considerations, such as the use of shared sleep spaces or makeshift bedding, with the influence of communal living arrangements or resource constraints.

Sleep practices often intertwine with **cultural rituals and routines**. In many Mediterranean and Latin American cultures, the concept of the siesta embodies a cultural tradition of taking a midday break for rest. This practice not only involves a physical space for napping but also encompasses social and cultural norms surrounding rest and relaxation. People often integrate the siesta into their daily lives, with businesses and schools adjusting their schedules to accommodate this period of rest.

In contrast, some **Asian cultures** may include sleep rituals such as herbal teas or meditation before bedtime to promote relaxation and restful sleep. Traditional Chinese medicine firmly assert the importance of establishing a calming pre-sleep routine to balance the body's energy and enhance sleep quality. This reflects a cultural understanding of sleep as part of a broader holistic approach to health.

The culture of sleep environments and practices illustrates how diverse cultural traditions, modern conveniences and social factors shape our approach to rest. From traditional sleeping arrangements to contemporary sleep hygiene practices; these cultural attitudes emphasize the complex interplay between environment, rituals, and individual well-being.

SLEEP RITUALS AND BELIEFS

Sleep rituals and beliefs have deep roots in cultural practices and reflect a society's understanding of rest, health, and the supernatural. These rituals shape how different cultures approach sleep by integrating spiritual, social, and practical elements into the act of resting.

In many ancient and traditional cultures, sleep was a time for connection with the spiritual world or a means of receiving guidance from deities or ancestors, as seen in ancient Egypt. It served as a form of divine communication. The Egyptians believed that dreams were messages from the gods and that the quality of sleep could reflect one's spiritual state. Temples and priests played a key role in interpreting dreams and providing guidance based on these nocturnal visions.

Similarly, people in ancient Greece saw dreams as omens or messages from the divine, and they usually performed rituals and prayers to seek favourable dreams or protect themselves from nightmares. Religious and philosophical thoughts deeply integrate sleep, reflecting a belief in the connection between rest and divinity.

Many Indigenous cultures in North America place view dreams as powerful sources of wisdom and spiritual insight. The Ojibwe (Chippewa) people, the largest indigenous Indian group north of Mexico, believe that dreamcatchers filter out bad dreams while allowing only positive ones to pass through. The practice of hanging these handmade objects above sleeping areas reflects their cultural belief in protecting and guiding one's sleep experience.

In many African cultures, particularly in Western Africa, communal sleeping arrangements and shared bedtime stories form part of nightly rituals that strengthen social bonds and impart cultural values. The belief that social harmony and communal support deeply influence sleep underscores the role of sleep as a shared cultural experience.

In contemporary societies, sleep rituals often reflect a blend of traditional practices and modern scientific understanding. Many people engage in pre-sleep routines designed to promote relaxation and improve sleep quality, such as reading, taking warm baths, or practicing mindfulness. The growing awareness of sleep hygiene and the importance of creating a restful environment significantly influences these sleep rituals.

For example, the use of technology to enhance sleep, such as sleep-tracking devices or white noise machines, represents a modern approach to managing and understanding sleep. While scientific research grounds these practices, they also reflect cultural values surrounding the pursuit of optimal health and well-being.

Cultural beliefs also influence how people perceive and respond to sleep disturbances, such as nightmares. In some cultures, people perceive nightmares as omens or signs of spiritual distress. Ritualistic cleansing ceremonies or specific prayers are employed to ward off negative influences and to address these sleep disturbances. In contrast, many Western cultures often approach sleep disturbances from a medical perspective, emphasizing the diagnosis and treatment of underlying conditions. This approach reflects a cultural belief in addressing sleep issues through scientific and clinical means rather than through spiritual or communal practices.

THE IMPACT OF MODERNISATION

The impact of modernization on the culture of sleep is profound and significant. It is reshaping how people approach rest, sleep environments, and daily routines. As societies have transitioned from agrarian to industrial and now to digital economies, the culture of sleep has evolved in response to technological advancements, changing work patterns, and new social norms.

Modernization has introduced a range of technologies that have transformed sleep practices and environments. The advent of electric lighting has extended the day well beyond natural light, eventually leading to shifts in sleep patterns. With artificial light, people began to stay awake longer, thereby altering the natural circadian rhythm that previously aligned with the rising and setting of the sun. This shift has led to the phenomenon of "social jetlag," where individuals struggle to synchronize their internal clocks with societal schedules.

Additionally, modern technology has brought innovations such as sleep-tracking devices and apps, which provide insights into sleep patterns and quality. While these tools can help people optimize their sleep, they also introduce new pressures and anxieties about achieving "perfect" sleep. The focus on quantifying and optimizing sleep reflects a cultural shift towards managing and controlling various aspects of life, including rest.

The transition from agrarian to industrial societies brought about significant changes in work patterns, which continue to influence sleep culture. In industrialized societies, the rigid 9-to-5 workday, has become the established norm that standardizes sleep schedule for many individuals.

However, as economies have shifted towards service and technology sectors, irregular and shift work have become more prevalent. These changes have led to the rise of shift work disorder and other sleep-related challenges as individuals struggle to adapt their sleep patterns to unconventional working hours.

The modern emphasis on productivity and constant connectivity has significantly affected sleep. The pressure to work long hours and remain accessible beyond traditional working hours can result in sleep deprivation. The culture of "hustle" and the glorification of busyness, often prioritize work over rest, ultimately contributing to widespread sleep issues and an increasing awareness of the need for better sleep management.

Urbanization has also transformed living conditions and sleep environments. In densely populated urban areas, individuals often reside in smaller spaces with limited privacy, which can affect sleep quality.

Noise pollution, light pollution and overcrowding are prevalent issues in cities that hinder the ability to achieve restful sleep.

Modern homes are equipped with various amenities designed to enhance comfort, such as temperature control systems, high-quality mattresses, and blackout curtains. These advancements reflect the cultural shift toward creating an ideal sleep environment that caters to individual preferences and improving sleep quality.

Modernization has also influenced cultural attitudes towards sleep hygiene and wellness. There is a growing recognition of the importance of sleep for overall health, driven by scientific research and public health campaigns. Concepts such as "sleep hygiene" and "sleep wellness" emphasize practices like maintaining a consistent sleep schedule, creating a restful environment, and avoiding stimulants before bedtime.

These practices reflect a shift towards a proactive approach to health and self-care.

Globalization has facilitated the exchange of cultural practices and attitudes towards sleep. The Western focus on sleep hygiene and technology has influenced sleep practices in other cultures, leading to a blend of traditional and modern approaches. Conversely, practices from other cultures, such as the Japanese concept of "inemuri" (sleeping in public), have gained recognition and influence in Western societies.

The rise of social media and digital communication has introduced new dynamics that affect sleep culture. The constant connectivity enabled by smartphones and social media can lead to "social media insomnia," where individuals struggle to fall asleep due to excessive screen time or anxiety about online interactions. The presence of screens in the bedroom and the habit of checking notifications before bed can disrupt sleep patterns and hinder the ability to achieve restful sleep.

THE IMPACT OF GOVERNMENT POLICIES AND SUPPORT

Government policies significantly shape the culture of sleep. These policies influence sleep patterns, public health and societal norms through regulations, workplace standardization, and public health initiatives. These policies can affect everything from work hours to school schedules, and their effects permeate various aspects of daily life.

One of the most direct ways that government policies influence sleep culture is through workplace regulations. Labour laws and regulations establish standards for work hours, breaks, and overtime, which directly affect sleep patterns.

Regulations that limit maximum work hours can help prevent excessive work-related fatigue. Policies ensuring that workers receive sufficient rest between shifts and prohibiting excessive overtime can very well contribute to better sleep hygiene and overall health.

In many countries, policymakers design regulations to manage shift work and night shifts to mitigate the negative effects of irregular sleep patterns on workers' health. Policies requiring employers to provide adequate rest breaks and manage shift rotations can help reduce the risk of shift work disorder and enhance sleep quality.

Government policies related to school start times and educational schedules influence sleep culture, particularly among children and adolescents. Policies regarding school start times can affect students' sleep patterns. Research has shown that later school start times can lead to improved sleep duration and quality among teenagers. In response to these findings, some governments and school districts have adjusted start times to better align with adolescents' natural sleep patterns.

Additionally, policies regarding the amount of homework and the scheduling of extracurricular activities can also affect students' sleep. Limiting homework and balancing extracurricular activities with adequate rest is crucial for maintaining students' overall health and well-being.

Government-led public health initiatives and campaigns play a vital role in shaping attitudes toward sleep and promoting healthy sleep practices.

Governments frequently sponsor sleep education programs to raise awareness about the significance of sleep and offer guidance on healthy sleep habits. These initiatives aim to inform the public on topics such as sleep hygiene, the effects of sleep deprivation as well as strategies for enhancing sleep quality.

Funding for sleep research fosters the development of new insights into sleep disorders, treatments, and best practices. Government support for sleep research advances our understanding of sleep and helps reform policies and public health strategies.

Driving Regulations governing commercial drivers' hours of service and rest requirements aim to prevent drowsy driving and enhance road safety. These regulations acknowledge the impact of sleep deprivation on driving performance and public safety.

Occupational Safety Standards that address workplace safety, including guidelines for managing fatigue in high-risk jobs such as healthcare and emergency services, also contribute to maintaining safe working conditions and ensuring adequate rest for workers.

Policies that offer paid leave for illness or personal reasons can alleviate stress and enable individuals to prioritize their health, including their sleep. Access to paid sick leave ensures that individuals can take time off to recover from illnesses without financial strain, which can enhance sleep quality and overall health.

Economic support programs such as unemployment benefits or housing assistance can lessen financial stress and contribute to improved sleep. Financial stability allows individuals to concentrate on maintaining a healthy lifestyle, including obtaining sufficient rest.

Policies that ensure adequate housing conditions, including regulations on noise, insulation, and space, contribute to improved sleep environments. Access to quality housing can also affect sleep quality by providing a comfortable and safe space for rest.

Urban planning policies that address issues such as noise pollution, light pollution, and access to green spaces can also influence sleep. Establishing well-designed urban environments with minimal disruptions promotes relaxation and supports healthier sleep patterns.

THE IMPACT OF SLEEP AND WELLNESS MOVEMENTS

Health and wellness movements raise awareness about the importance of rest as well as the benefits of integrating sleep into the broader health and lifestyle practices. These movements have shifted cultural attitudes, influenced sleep practices and promoted new approaches to achieving better sleep quality.

Health and wellness movements play a crucial role in highlighting the importance of sleep for overall health. As these movements have gained traction, there has been a growing recognition of sleep as a vital component of well-being, on par with diet and exercise

Public health campaigns and educational programs have enhanced understanding of the benefits of adequate sleep and the risks associated with sleep deprivation. These campaigns often emphasize the impact of sleep on mental health, physical health, and cognitive function.

The focus on wellness has spurred interest in sleep research, leading to a deeper understanding of sleep disorders, sleep hygiene, and the physiological processes underlying sleep. The frequent sharing of research findings with the public greatly influences their attitudes and behaviours related to sleep.

Sleep has become an essential component of holistic wellness practices, reflecting a more comprehensive approach to health. Wellness movements have popularized the concept of sleep hygiene, which involves creating optimal conditions for restorative sleep. This includes practices such as maintaining a consistent sleep schedule, establishing a calming bedtime routine, and optimizing the sleep environment with blackout curtains, managing noise, and controlling room temperature.

The incorporation of mindfulness and relaxation techniques into wellness routines has also influenced sleep culture. Practices such as meditation, deep breathing exercises and progressive muscle relaxation are effective methods for reducing stress and enhance sleep quality.

Health and wellness movements have propelled the development and popularization of sleep-related technologies and products designed to improve sleep quality. The emergence of wearable sleep trackers and smartphone apps reflects a growing interest in monitoring and optimizing sleep. These technologies provide individuals with insights into their sleep patterns, helping them make informed decisions about their sleep habits and environments.

Innovations in sleep aids such as high-tech mattresses, adjustable beds, and sleep masks, have become increasingly accessible. These products offer innovative solutions to enhance sleep quality and address specific sleep challenges.

Cultural transformation towards recognizing rest and recovery as vital components of a healthy lifestyle contrasts with earlier cultural attitudes that often prioritized productivity and constant activity over sufficient rest.

The ideology of sleep as a crucial aspect of self-care is gaining traction, reflecting a wider cultural trend toward prioritizing personal well-being and incorporating self-care practices into daily routines.

Health and wellness movements have also highlighted sleep disorders and the necessity for effective management. Awareness of various sleep disorders such as insomnia, sleep apnea, and restless leg syndrome, has increased. Wellness movements have played a role in combating the stigmatization of these conditions and encouraging individuals to seek help and treatment.

Advocacy efforts within the wellness community have resulted in increased support for research, treatment, and resources related to sleep disorders, including promoting access to healthcare professionals specializing in sleep medicine and encouraging early intervention.

The incorporation of sleep into workplace wellness programs highlights the influence of health and wellness movements on professional settings.

Numerous organizations now include sleep as a key element of workplace wellness programs, acknowledging the effect of sleep on employee health, productivity, and performance. Initiatives may involve providing resources on sleep hygiene, offering flexible work schedules, or establishing quiet areas for rest.

The focus on wellness has shaped corporate culture, with some companies implementing policies that promote work-life balance and employee well-being. This includes recognizing the significance of adequate rest to enable employees to manage their sleep needs more effectively.

SLEEP NEEDS

The quest to completely appreciate and understand sleep is a never-ending pursuit that recognizes sleep is not a fixed, universal experience. Factors like age, lifestyle, health, and even genetic makeup, shape up individual sleep requirements, thereby rendering the science of sleep as varied as the individuals who experience it.

While sleep experts propose that adults should aim for 7-9 hours of sleep each night, the truth is, your ideal amount of sufficient sleep may fall outside of this range and that is okay. The key is to listen to your body and its signals.

From the moment we are born, our sleep requirements shift and change as we grow. A newborn, small and new to the world, might need up to 17 hours of sleep a day, while a teenager, navigating the highs and lows of adolescence, needs somewhere between 8 and 10 hours. As we reach adulthood, that number tends to settle between 7 and 9 hours. Yet, as we age, something interesting happens: older adults may find they do not need as much sleep, though they often experience a decline in the quality of their rest. It is almost as if each stage of life comes with its own rhythm and pattern of rest and comprehensively understanding these rhythms and sleep patterns can be the first step towards figuring out your own sleep needs.

Age is not the only factor at play. Some people spring out of bed fully refreshed after just six hours of sleep, while others may drag through the day if they do not get a solid nine. Sleep needs are as personal as your fingerprints. That is why rigidly adhering to a prescribed number of hours can sometimes do more harm than good. Instead, try this: pay attention to how you feel during the day. Are you alert, focused, and clear-headed, or are you slogging through, groggy and irritable. Your daytime energy and mood are clues that reveal whether you are getting the deep sleep that your body craves.

Then there is the matter of lifestyle. If you are an athlete pushing your body to its physical limits, you may need more sleep to recover and repair your muscles. Alternatively, if you are navigating a particularly stressful period in your life, such as dealing with stress or illness, both can demand more from your body, and that demand often shows up in your sleep patterns. During these times, your body may call out for extra rest, urging you to slow down and create the space needed to heal and reset.

Quantity, however, is only half the story. It is not just about how long you sleep but how well you sleep. Imagine lying in bed for 8 hours, tossing and turning, your mind racing, your body never truly relaxing. Even if you hit the recommended number of hours, restless sleep or frequent waking can rob you of the deep, restorative stages of rest that your body so desperately needs. Without that deep sleep, it is as if you are running on an empty tank. So, yes, count your hours, but also pay attention to how you feel when you wake up.

Of course, life sometimes gets in the way. There are late nights, early mornings, and times when sleep, simply is not a priority. When that happens, you might try to "catch up" by sleeping in on the weekend. While that extra rest can help a little, it does not quite erase the effects of sleep deprivation. No matter how many hours you sleep in on Saturday, you cannot make up for the long-term neglect of your sleep in a single night. Consistency is what counts most.

At the heart of it all, the answer lies within you. Your body is always sending signals, letting you know if you have had enough rest or if you are running on empty. If you wake up feeling refreshed, alert, and ready to take on the day, you are likely on the right track. However, if you find yourself reaching for that extra cup of coffee just to stay awake, or if you find yourself dragging through the afternoon, it might be time to rethink your sleep habits.

In the end, understanding your sleep needs is about more than just hours. The quality of your rest depends on the efficacy of your energy, stability of your mood, as well as the clarity of your thoughts throughout each day. By tuning in to what your body is telling you and making sleep a priority, you can create a routine that allows you not just to function, but truly thrive.

CAUSES OF VARIATIONS IN SLEEP NEEDS AND DURATION

Imagine a room full of people, each with their own unique sleep patterns and needs. Some may wake up refreshed after just six hours of rest, while others need a full ten hours to feel truly recharged. This is because sleep needs are not the same for everyone due to a number of variations that shape how much rest each person requires.

Though we often hear that adults need seven to nine hours of sleep, the reality is far more complex. Age, genetics, lifestyle, and overall health all play a role in determining how much sleep we need to function at our best. While one person might be able to power through the day with minimal rest, another may struggle without a longer night of sleep. These natural differences remind us that sleep is an individual experience, shaped by our unique bodies and minds. These unique variables interact in complex ways, shaping how much sleep we require at different stages of life and how our sleep patterns evolve over time.

These variables include:

1
Biological Rhythms:
The Role of the Circadian Clock

The body's internal clock, known as the circadian rhythm, plays a vital role in regulating sleep-wake cycles. At its core is the hypothalamus, a small region in the brain that responds to light and darkness. This circadian clock influences when we feel sleepy and when we are most alert, largely determining our sleep patterns.

Exposure to natural light during the day helps regulate the circadian rhythm, promoting wakefulness during daylight hours and sleepiness at night. In contrast, artificial light, particularly blue light from screens, can disrupt this rhythm, delaying the release of melatonin, the hormone responsible for signalling sleep.

As we age, melatonin production changes, affecting our sleep patterns. For example, teenagers often experience a delayed release of melatonin, leading to late sleep times, while older adults may produce less melatonin, contributing to earlier bedtimes and more fragmented sleep.

The circadian clock regulates various physiological processes over a roughly 24-hour cycle. It is a key player in maintaining the body's balance and plays a crucial role in determining the timing of sleep, the quality of rest, and overall well-being.

At the heart of the circadian rhythm is a group of cells in the brain called the **suprachiasmatic nucleus (SCN),** located in the hypothalamus. This "master clock" coordinates daily cycles of activity across the body, synchronizing them to external cues, most notably light and darkness. The **SCN** receives signals from the eyes about light exposure and uses this information to regulate the production of melatonin, a hormone that helps induce sleep.

Light exposure in the morning signals the body to wake up, suppressing melatonin production, while the onset of darkness triggers the **SCN** to increase melatonin levels, making us feel sleepy. This interaction between the circadian clock and external environmental cues is a result of brainwave **entrainment.** This is due to the observation that our internal timekeeping is constantly adjusting to the environment, ensuring that we remain aligned with the day-night cycle.

The circadian rhythm extends beyond sleep and wakefulness: it also regulates body temperature, hormone release, digestion, and energy levels. For example, body temperature tends to peak during the day, enhancing alertness, and drops in the evening, signalling the body to wind down for rest.

The circadian clock acts as our body's natural sleep regulator that determines when we feel the strongest need to sleep and wake up. It interacts with another process, called **sleep pressure** or the **homeostatic sleep drive**, which builds up the longer we are awake. Together, these two systems ensure that we not only fall asleep but also maintain consistent, healthy sleep patterns over time.

When our circadian rhythm aligns harmoniously with our environment, we can sleep and wake according to natural light cycles, thereby experiencing better sleep quality. However, disruptions to the circadian clock, such as shift work, jet lag, or excessive exposure to artificial light at night, can lead to misaligned sleep-wake cycles. This misalignment can result in sleep difficulties, decreased energy levels, and impaired cognitive function.

2
Lifestyle Choices:
The Impact of Daily Habits

Imagine how the decisions we make each day shape the ways and duration of our sleep. Our lifestyle choices, including how we move, eat, and manage stress, to the routines we follow and the technology we use, all play a significant role in determining how much rest we get and how refreshed we feel. These choices affect not only how easily we fall asleep but also the quality of our rest, setting the tone for how our bodies recover and recharge.

Take physical activity, for example. A brisk walk or workout can help us fall asleep faster and enjoy deeper, restorative sleep. However, timing is important because, exercising right before bed can create the opposite effect, thereby making it harder to wind down as our bodies are still buzzing with energy. On the other hand, a light yoga session or gentle stretching in the evening can help calm the body and prepare it for rest.

What we eat also matters. Taking large meals, spicy foods, and caffeine closer to bedtime can disrupt sleep. Caffeine is a well-known stimulant that can keep us awake for hours, while alcohol, although it may initially make us drowsy, interferes with deep sleep and often leads to frequent awakenings. Staying hydrated is essential, but drinking too much water before bed can result in restless nights filled with trips to the bathroom. Choosing lighter, sleep-friendly foods in the evening can make it easier to drift off and stay asleep.

Stress is another powerful force that impacts sleep. High levels of anxiety can keep our minds racing long after the day is done, preventing us from falling or staying asleep. How we manage stress, whether through meditation, deep breathing, or simply setting aside time to unwind, can make a huge difference. Establishing a calming bedtime routine signals to the brain that it is time to relax, paving the way for a smoother transition into sleep.

Even our work schedules also play a part. People who work irregular hours or night shifts often find their sleep patterns disrupted because their internal clocks are out of synchronisation with the natural rhythms of day and night. For those with regular 9-to-5 jobs, long work hours or social obligations can still cut into precious sleep time, leading to chronic sleep deprivation. Keeping a consistent sleep schedule, even on weekends, helps maintain a healthy sleep cycle, ensuring that we get enough rest to function at our best.

3
Environmental Conditions: The Role of the Surroundings

Environmental conditions play a pivotal role in shaping both the quality and duration of our sleep. The spaces we sleep in, along with external stimuli, can either create an environment conducive to deep, restorative rest or one that leads to frequent disturbances and poor sleep. Factors like light, noise, temperature, air quality, and even bedding contribute to how well we sleep each night.

Noise is one of the most disruptive environmental factors. Even low levels of background noise can cause the brain to remain partially alert, preventing deep sleep or causing frequent awakenings throughout the night. This disruption affects both the quality and duration of sleep, often resulting in daytime fatigue and impaired cognitive function.

Different types of noise—from street traffic to a partner snoring or even the hum of household appliances can disturb sleep. Sudden or intermittent noises are particularly disruptive, as they trigger the startle response and lead to brief awakenings or lighter sleep. Over time, chronic noise exposure reduces sleep efficiency, making it harder to achieve the restorative rest essential for physical and mental recovery.

One way to mitigate the effects of noise is by using white noise machines or earplugs to mask disruptive sounds. White noise machine provides a consistent auditory backdrop that drowns out sudden changes in sound levels, allowing for more uninterrupted sleep.

The temperature of our sleep environment also plays a critical role in sleep regulation. The body's core temperature naturally drops in preparation for sleep, and maintaining a cool room helps facilitate this process. Sleep experts recommend keeping the room between 60°F to 67°F (15°C to 19°C) for optimal sleep, as temperatures that are too high or too low can lead to discomfort and disrupt sleep cycles.

When the room is too warm, it becomes difficult for the body to cool down, resulting in restless sleep and frequent awakenings, which can prevent deeper stages of sleep like REM and slow-wave sleep. Overheating during sleep has also been associated with vivid dreams or nightmares. The heat can intensify brain activity during the REM stage of sleep, where most dreaming occurs. This heightened activity, combined with the body's response to illness, can lead to vivid, often bizarre, and sometimes unsettling dreams.

On the other hand, a very cold room forces the body to work harder to maintain its core temperature, which can lead to disrupted sleep. Adjusting the thermostat, using breathable bedding, or adding a fan can help regulate room temperature for better rest.

Air quality is another critical factor that affects sleep. Poor air quality— whether due to allergens, dust, or lack of ventilation, can lead to breathing difficulties during sleep. This is especially true for individuals with respiratory conditions like asthma, sleep apnea, or allergies, which may escalate due to poor indoor air quality.

Exposure to airborne irritants can cause nasal congestion, coughing, or throat irritation, all of which can disrupt sleep. Keeping the air clean by using air purifiers, frequently changing bedding, and ensuring good ventilation helps reduce allergens and improve breathing at night.

Extremely dry air can irritate the respiratory system, while overly humid environments can promote the growth of mould and dust mites, both of which can trigger allergic reactions. Using a humidifier or dehumidifier to maintain optimal humidity levels (between 30% and 50%) can create a healthier sleep environment.

The physical comfort of your sleep environment including your mattress, pillows, and bedding can directly affect how well you sleep. An unsupportive mattress that is too firm or too soft can lead to discomfort, poor spinal alignment, and sleep disruptions. Over time, an unsupportive sleep surface can cause back pain or stiffness, making it harder to get a full night's rest.

Choosing the right mattress and pillows that suit your sleep preferences and body type is essential for gaining quality sleep. For instance, some people may benefit from memory foam mattresses that contour to the body's shape, while others might prefer firmer mattresses for better support. Pillows should provide adequate support for the neck and head, thereby promoting spinal alignment and reducing strain.

In addition to the texture of sleep surfaces bedding materials can also influence sleep. Breathable, natural fibres like cotton or linen help regulate body temperature by wicking away moisture and allowing ventilation by reducing the chance of overheating. Comfortable, high-quality bedding makes the sleep environment more inviting, encouraging longer, uninterrupted sleep.

The layout and organisation of the sleep environment also contribute to sleep quality. A cluttered, chaotic bedroom can create a sense of uneasiness, making it difficult to relax and fall asleep. The brain associates clutter with stress and unfinished tasks, which can keep the mind engaged rather than allowing it to wind down.

Creating a minimalist, calming bedroom environment that is free from unnecessary distractions can help foster a sense of peace and relaxation. Keeping the bedroom space clean and organized as well as designating it primarily for sleep, helps the brain associate the bedroom with rest. This includes minimizing the presence of work materials, electronics, or bright screens, which can cause mental overstimulation and keep the mind active when it should be winding down.

Certain scents help promote relaxation and improve sleep quality. Aromatherapy, particularly with essential oils like lavender, chamomile, or jasmine essential oils, is good for reducing anxiety and promoting better sleep. Using essential oil diffusers, scented candles, or aromatherapy pillows infused with relaxing aroma scents trigger a relaxation response in the brain, making it easier to fall asleep and stay asleep

4
Health Conditions:
The Impact of Physical and Mental Health

Sleep quality and duration closely relate to physical and mental health, with each affecting the other in a continuous cycle. Poor sleep can lead to deteriorating health, while issues with physical and mental health can disrupt sleep patterns.

Physical health encompasses a wide range of factors, including chronic medical conditions, pain, medication use, and overall fitness levels. Each of these can directly affect how well we sleep.

Chronic conditions such as diabetes, heart disease, asthma, and arthritis can interfere with sleep. For example, individuals with diabetes may experience fluctuations in blood sugar levels that disrupt sleep, while those with heart conditions might experience sleep apnea, a condition where breathing repeatedly stops and starts during sleep. Asthma can cause nighttime awakenings due to difficulty breathing, and arthritis can lead to pain that makes it challenging to find a comfortable sleeping position.

Chronic pain conditions, including back pain, fibromyalgia, and joint pain, can severely affect sleep quality. Physical discomfort can make it difficult to fall asleep or stay asleep, leading to fragmented rest and reduction in overall sleep duration. The body's need to manage pain often takes precedence over the need for restorative sleep, thereby creating a vicious cycle in which poor sleep exacerbates pain sensitivity and increases discomfort.

Hormonal imbalances can also affect sleep quality. Conditions like hypothyroidism and hyperthyroidism, which involve a deficiency or excess of a hormones produced by the butterfly-shaped thyroid gland in the neck, can disrupt heart rate, body temperature, and various metabolic processes. Hypothyroidism is mostly prevalent in older women.

Hormonal changes during the menstrual cycle or menopause can also disrupt sleep patterns. For example, many women experience sleep disturbances due to fluctuations in oestrogen and progesterone levels, which can affect mood and contribute to insomnia or nighttime awakenings.

Regular physical activity is crucial for maintaining physical health and has a significant impact on sleep. Exercise can help regulate sleep patterns by promoting deeper sleep. Conversely, a sedentary lifestyle can lead to weight gain, which may negatively affect sleep. Maintaining a balanced exercise routine supports overall health and better sleep quality.

Mental health is another critical factor that significantly affects sleep. Conditions like anxiety, depression, and stress can lead to insomnia, while poor sleep can further exacerbate these mental health issues.

Anxiety is one of the most common mental health issues linked to sleep disturbances. Individuals with anxiety disorders often struggle to relax, making it difficult to fall asleep. The racing thoughts and heightened arousal associated with anxiety can lead to prolonged sleep onset times and fragmented sleep. Additionally, anxiety can cause physical symptoms, such as increased heart rate or muscle tension, further disrupting sleep.

Depression is another mental health condition with a complex relationship to sleep. Some individuals may experience hypersomnia, or excessive sleepiness, while others may struggle with insomnia. Those with depression often find it challenging to maintain a consistent sleep schedule, leading to irregular sleep patterns. This relationship is bidirectional: poor sleep can worsen depression symptoms, while depression can make sleep more difficult.

Stress, whether acute or chronic, significantly affects sleep quality. High stress levels activate the body's fight-or-flight response, increasing cortisol levels, which disrupt sleep cycles and hinder relaxation. This can create a constant state of hyperarousal, making it hard to wind down and fall asleep.

Certain medications can also affect sleep quality and duration. For instance, some antidepressants may cause drowsiness, while others may lead to insomnia as a side effect. Medications for high blood pressure or asthma can interfere with sleep patterns as well. Understanding the potential effects of prescribed medications is crucial for effectively managing sleep quality.

The interplay between sleep quality and physical and mental health can create a vicious cycle. Poor sleep can exacerbate physical health issues and mental health disorders, leading to increased fatigue, irritability, and decreased overall quality of life. Conversely, health issues can lead to poor sleep, resulting in a feedback loop that is difficult to break.

For example, individuals with chronic pain may find it hard to sleep well, which can increase their pain sensitivity and exacerbate their condition. Likewise, those experiencing high levels of stress or anxiety may struggle to sleep, leading to increased irritability and difficulty coping with daily challenges.

5
Developmental Stages

The onset of sleep cycles in infancy marks a fascinating phase in a baby's development, which reflects their body's growing ability to regulate sleep patterns. In the first few months of life, infants lack a mature sleep-wake cycle, resulting in shorter sleep periods predominantly composed of Rapid Eye Movement (REM) sleep. This type of sleep is crucial for brain development, aiding in the formation of neural connections and sensory processing.

New-borns typically require 14 to 17 hours of sleep per day, occurring in short bursts rather than long stretches. Their underdeveloped circadian rhythms and need for frequent feeding influence this pattern. They do not yet have distinct day and night sleep patterns and may sleep anywhere from two to four hours at a time, and waking frequently to feed. This irregularity stems from their small stomach size, which necessitates regular feeding, along with their immature circadian rhythm—the internal biological clock that regulates sleep and wakefulness.

As infants grow, their sleep begins to consolidate, allowing for longer periods at nighttime sleep and fewer daytime naps. By their first year, most babies sleep through the night with one or two daytime naps, indicating the emergence of more structured sleep patterns.

These early stages of sleep cycle development are foundational for the child's overall growth, supporting everything from brain development to physical health. As their sleep becomes more consolidated and predictable, so too does their ability to engage more actively with the world during their waking hours.

Establishing sleep routine in childhood is crucial for a child's development and overall wellbeing. From their earliest stages, children thrive on predictability. Although the need for sleep gradually decreases as they grow, it remains high during childhood. Toddlers typically require 11 to 14 hours of sleep per day, including one or two naps.

As children enter preschool age, their sleep patterns become more consolidated, with most dropping naps altogether and sleeping 10 to 13 hours at night. Parents can help by setting consistent bedtimes and wake-up times. This regularity helps signal to the child's body that it is time to wind down and prepare for rest when the time comes. Common bedtime rituals, such as a warm bath, a bedtime story, or quiet play, help indicate that the day is ending and sleep is approaching. Creating a calm, soothing environment along with dim lighting, can help encourage relaxation.

Sleep during childhood is vital for physical growth, cognitive development, and emotional regulation. During periods of rapid growth, the body places greater emphasis on deep sleep stages (slow-wave sleep) to meet its restorative needs.

The sleep patterns established during these formative years have a lasting impact, not only aiding in physical development but also laying the foundation for healthy sleep habits in adolescence and adulthood. Consistency, patience, and a nurturing environment where the child feels safe and comfortable are key to establishing a successful sleep routine.

The shift in sleep patterns during adolescence brings significant changes in sleep needs and patterns, influenced by both biological and social factors. Teenagers typically require about 8 to 10 hours of sleep each night, but many experience a shift in their circadian rhythms, resulting in a natural tendency to stay up late and wake up later. This delay in sleep timing, known as "delayed sleep phase," occurs due to hormonal changes, particularly the later release of melatonin during puberty.

Sleep deprivation during this stage can adversely affect mood, cognitive function, and overall health, making it essential for teens to prioritize sleep despite the demands of their busy lives. Lack of sleep can lead to irritability, difficulty concentrating, and an increased risk of mental health issues such as anxiety and depression. Additionally, physical consequences like weakened immune function and impaired motor skills may become common.

Despite these challenges, sleep routines during adolescence can still be under support and supervision. Encouraging consistent bedtimes, reducing exposure to screens before sleep (since blue light can interfere with melatonin production), and creating a quiet, dark sleep environment can help mitigate the effects of this biological shift. However, societal and academic pressures often make it difficult for teens to align their schedules with their body's natural sleep needs.

In adulthood, the challenge of balancing sleep with increasing responsibilities becomes more regular. As individuals transition into their 20s and 30s, the demands of work, family, social obligations, and personal pursuits often compete for time, pushing sleep lower on the priority list.

Most adults need around 7 to 9 hours of sleep per night, yet many find themselves chronically sleep-deprived due to work deadlines, parenting, or social commitments. This sleep deprivation can quickly compound, leading to fatigue, decreased productivity, irritability and even health issues like weakened immunity, weight gain, and an increased risk of chronic conditions like diabetes and cardiovascular disease. While the required amount of sleep can vary based on lifestyle, health, and genetics, young adults may still feel the residual effects of the delayed sleep phase, often referred to as being a "night owl," with many gradually shifting to earlier sleep times as they age.

Balancing work, family and social responsibilities to achieve sufficient sleep remains a significant challenge for adults. The pressures of modern life, including long work hours, commuting and constant digital connectivity, contribute to sleep deprivation. Prioritizing sleep and maintaining good sleep hygiene are essential for sustaining physical health, cognitive function and emotional well-being.

Recognising sleep as a non-negotiable aspect of self-care allows adults to recharge both physically and mentally, leading to more balanced and sustainable approaches to managing the demands of everyday life.

As people age, natural changes in sleep architecture and patterns occur. Older adults may still require about 7 to 8 hours of sleep, but they often experience lighter sleep with more frequent awakenings throughout the night. The amount of deep sleep (slow-wave sleep) decreases, while the time spent in lighter sleep stages increases, making older adults more vulnerable to disturbances and leading to feelings of being less refreshed upon waking.

Additionally, older adults may experience a shift toward earlier bedtimes and wake times, known as "advanced sleep phase." This shift is partly due to changes in the body's internal clock and a reduction in melatonin production.

Other factors, such as medical conditions, medications, and decreased physical activity, can also influence sleep in older adults. It is important for them to focus on creating a conducive sleep environment, maintaining a regular sleep schedule and addressing any underlying health issues that may affect sleep quality.

PRINCIPLES OF GOOD SLEEP
1
PRIORITIZING YOUR SLEEP

Prioritizing sleep means recognizing it as a fundamental pillar of your health and well-being and giving it the importance it deserves in your daily routine. Imagine treating sleep as non-negotiable—something as essential as eating or breathing—because it truly is. When you prioritize sleep, you set yourself up for better health, improved mood, and greater productivity.

Here is how you can make sleep a top priority in your life:

First, it is essential to recognize the value of sleep. Sleep is not just downtime; it is when your body and mind repair and recharge. During sleep, your brain processes information, your immune system strengthens, and your body restores its energy reserves. By placing sleep at the top of your priority list, you are investing in your long-term health and well-being.

Start by establishing a consistent sleep schedule. Just like any other important routine, your body thrives on regularity. Go to bed and wake up at the same time every day, even on weekends. This consistency strengthens your internal clock, making it easier to fall asleep at night and wake up feeling refreshed.

Next, you will need to set boundaries around your sleep time. In today's busy world, it is easy to let work, social activities, or screen time encroach on your rest. Nevertheless, when sleep is a priority, it becomes a sacred time that you protect. Create a "no-excuses" policy for getting to bed on time, even if it means saying no to late-night work emails or endless scrolling on social media.

Another crucial step is to create an environment that supports sleep. Your bedroom should be a place of rest, free from distractions and disruptions. Make your sleep space as comfortable as possible—cool, quiet, and dark. Use blackout curtains, white noise machines, or whatever tools you need to create a peaceful environment that encourages deep, restful sleep. If life gets hectic, it can be tempting to sacrifice sleep to fit more into your day. However, when you prioritize sleep, you realize that cutting corners on rest only hurts your productivity in the end. Stop viewing sleep as expendable; instead, see it as a critical component of your success—whether in your career, relationships, or personal well-being. Adequate sleep leads to better focus, creativity, and resilience.

It is also essential to plan your day around your sleep, not the other way around. This means setting up your daily schedule in a way that allows for plenty of time to wind down in the evening. Give yourself a buffer zone before bed—an hour or so to relax and transition from the day's activities. Whether it is reading, meditating, or taking a warm bath, these calming routines help signal to your body that it is time to sleep.

While prioritizing sleep, it is important to be mindful of your lifestyle choices. Things like diet, exercise, and stress management play significant roles in your sleep quality. Avoid heavy meals, caffeine, and alcohol too close to bedtime, and aim for regular physical activity, but not too late in the day. Managing stress through techniques like mindfulness or deep breathing can also ensure that you are not carrying the tension of the day into bed.

By prioritizing sleep, you will also learn to listen to your body. When you feel tired, honour that signal and allow yourself to rest. This might mean taking short naps during the day if needed or adjusting your schedule to ensure you are getting enough rest. Ignoring signs of fatigue only leads to burnout and negatively affects your health.

Finally, remember that prioritizing sleep is a form of self-care. As the world glorifies hustle and productivity, choosing to rest might feel like a radical act. Nevertheless, when you make sleep a priority, you are choosing to take care of yourself mentally, physically, and emotionally. You are giving your body the time it needs to heal, grow, and thrive.

By consciously prioritizing sleep, you are making a powerful statement that your health and well-being matter. In the end, this commitment to rest will lead to a more balanced, energized, and fulfilling life. Sleep is not a luxury but a necessity, and when you treat it as such, everything else in your life reaps the benefits.

2
PERSONALISING YOUR SLEEP

Personalizing your sleep is about tuning into your own body and creating an environment and routine that suits your unique needs. Imagine waking up every morning feeling refreshed and energized, knowing that your sleep schedule aligns perfectly with your natural rhythm.

To start, it is important to understand your body's natural inclination to sleep at a certain time. This will reveal whether you are naturally a morning person who thrives with early bedtimes or more of a night owl who does your best thinking as the world winds down. Knowing when your body is naturally wired to sleep can help you structure your day in harmony with your internal clock.

Next, figure out your ideal sleep duration. While seven to nine hours is a good general guideline, everyone's needs are different. You might require slightly more or less sleep to feel fully rested. Pay attention to how you feel after varying amounts of sleep, and adjust your routine gradually until you find what makes you feel your best.

However, it is not about just how long you sleep but also where you sleep. Creating a personalized sleep environment means turning your bedroom into a sleep sanctuary. Whether that means lowering the temperature to a cool, cosy level, choosing the perfect mattress, or controlling the light and sound, what works for one person might not work for another. Experiment until your surroundings feel just right.

The way you unwind at the end of the day is also important. Tailor your pre-sleep routine to your needs. For some, relaxing with a book or meditating can help quiet the mind. Others might need to avoid caffeine or heavy meals in the evening to drift off easily. The key is to create a ritual that signals to your body that it is time to slow down and prepare for rest.

It is also essential to recognize any personal sleep disruptors. Perhaps a heavy dinner keeps you awake, or exercising too late in the evening makes it hard to settle down. Fine-tune these factors by observing how your lifestyle choices affect your sleep.

For those who love data, technology can be a great ally in personalizing your sleep. With sleep trackers, you can monitor how much deep and Rapid Eye Movement (REM) sleep you are getting, and smart alarms can even wake you at the optimal time during your sleep cycle.

If you face unique challenges, such as sleep disorders, personalizing your sleep becomes even more important. Remember to synchronize your sleep with your daily life. If you have a flexible schedule, consider adjusting your sleep time to match your body's rhythm or incorporating naps to recharge. Managing stress is also key—whether it is through yoga, journaling, or other calming practices before bed, finding what works for you will make a big difference in your sleep quality.

By paying attention to your body's needs, environment, and routines, you can create a personalized approach to sleep that not only improves your rest but also enhances your overall well-being.

3
TRUSTING YOUR SLEEP

Trusting sleep is about letting go of the need to control or worry about it and believing in your body's natural ability to restore itself. Imagine approaching bedtime with a sense of calm, knowing that your body understands exactly what it needs to rest and recover. By shifting your mindset, you can allow sleep to come naturally and easily, without anxiety or overthinking.

To start, it is important to release the sleep anxiety that often creeps in when you cannot fall asleep or worry about how much rest you will get. By creating a peaceful environment and a calming routine, you set the stage for your body to do what it naturally does effortlessly—sleeping deeply. Instead of stressing, trust that your body will take care of it.

Part of this trust comes from understanding that sleep does not always follow a perfect pattern. Disruptions like waking up during the night or experiencing lighter sleep are normal. Trusting sleep means knowing that even if it is not perfect, your body is still benefiting. You are still resting, even during those moments when you are not asleep.

One of the simplest ways to trust sleep is to stop clock-watching. We have all been there—staring at the clock, calculating how many hours of sleep we are losing. This habit creates tension and makes it harder to sleep. Turn the clock away and focus on how your body feels. Trust that the time spent resting, whether you are asleep or not, is still valuable.

You also need to trust your body's signals. Your body knows when it is ready to sleep. Rather than forcing yourself to bed at a set time, tune into your body. When you feel sleepy, go to bed. By synchronizing with your body's natural rhythms, you will find it easier to fall asleep and wake up feeling refreshed.

It is also important to remember that your body is resilient. Even after a night of poor sleep, your body has ways to make up for the losses. It can increase the time spent in deep or Rapid Eye Movement (REM) sleep when you need it most. Trust that your body knows how to recover from lost sleep without you having to overthink or compensate.

When sleep is elusive, allow yourself to simply rest. Even if sleep does not come immediately, lying still in a relaxed state with your eyes closed is restorative. Trust that rest has its own benefits, and by focusing on relaxation rather than trying to force sleep, you give yourself the best chance of eventually drifting off.

Building confidence in your sleep routine is key. When you have established a consistent bedtime routine and created a sleep-friendly environment, you can let go of the pressure. You have done your part, and now it is time to trust that your body will take over from there.

Sleep will not always be perfect, and that is okay. Embrace imperfection and know that you do not need flawless sleep every single night to feel well-rested overall. Your body is adaptable, and occasional disturbances will not throw you off the balance. This mindset shift takes the pressure off and allows you to relax.

Most importantly, trusting sleep is about releasing control. Sleep is one of those things you cannot micromanage. It happens when you relax and allow it. Once you have set the right conditions—like a peaceful environment and a bedtime routine, it will naturally fall into place. Trust that your body knows exactly what to do and that sleep will come when it is ready.

Trust that even short or less-than-perfect nights of sleep are still contributing to your health. Over time, consistent rest adds up, and your body builds resilience. By trusting the process, you can find peace in knowing that sleep will always be there for you, naturally and effortlessly.

4
PROTECTING YOUR SLEEP

Protecting your sleep involves setting boundaries and creating habits that safeguard this essential part of your life. Imagine sleep as a precious resource—something that you need to shield from the chaos of daily life in order to function at your best. It is not just about how long you sleep, but how consistently you prioritize and protect that time.

One of the most important ways to protect your sleep is by establishing a routine. Going to bed and waking up at the same time every day, even on weekends, helps regulate your body's internal clock. This consistency sends a strong message to your brain that it is time to wind down and rest, making it easier to fall asleep and wake up refreshed.

Next, consider your pre-sleep environment. Is your bedroom quiet, dark, and cool? These are key elements that help you stay asleep throughout the night. Consider blackout curtains, a white noise machine, or even earplugs if necessary. Make your sleep space a sanctuary—somewhere you can retreat to for rest, free from distractions and disturbances.

Another critical aspect of protecting your sleep is what you do during the hours leading up to bedtime. Avoid stimulants like caffeine or nicotine in the late afternoon or evening, as they can interfere with your ability to fall asleep. Instead, engage in calming activities like reading, meditating, or gentle stretching to signal to your body that it is time to relax.

Limiting screen time is also essential. The blue light emitted from phones, tablets, and computers tricks your brain into thinking it is still daytime. Try to avoid screens at least an hour before bed, and if possible, set your phone to night mode to reduce blue light exposure.

Stress management is another major factor. Life is full of challenges, and it is easy for the worries of the day to follow you into bed. To protect your sleep, develop techniques to quiet your mind before you turning in. Journaling, deep breathing exercises, or progressive muscle relaxation can help reduce anxiety and clear your mind, making it easier to sleep soundly.

Your diet and exercise habits can also affect your sleep quality. While a balanced diet and regular exercise are great for your overall health, eating heavy meals late at night or exercising too close to bedtime can disrupt your sleep. Pay attention to how these factors affect you, and adjust your habits accordingly.

Finally, be mindful of sleep disruptors in your environment. If your job, family, or social life often cuts into your rest, set boundaries around your sleep schedule. Communicate your needs clearly to those around you, and be firm about keeping your sleep time sacred. Sometimes that means saying no to late-night plans or adjusting your routine to ensure you get the rest you need.

In the end, protecting your sleep is about prioritizing it as a vital part of your life. By creating a sleep-friendly environment, establishing a consistent routine, and making choices that promote rest, you can shield your sleep from the disruptions of daily life and enjoy the long-term benefits of deep, restorative rest.

INDICATORS OF POOR SLEEP

Poor sleep has a way of creeping into every corner of your life, often without you realizing it at first. While the signs may be subtle at times, they become unmistakable once you know what to look for. It often begins with a sense of daytime fatigue. Despite spending hours in bed, you feel like you are running on empty. You find yourself struggling to keep your eyes open during meetings, craving naps in the middle of the day, and needing that extra cup of coffee just to make it through.

However, it is not just about being tired. Concentration becomes a challenge as well. Tasks that used to be easy now feel overwhelming. You lose focus halfway through conversations, misplace items, or make mistakes at work. It is like a mental fog that will not lift, leaving you frustrated and less productive.

Then there is the shift in your mood. You might find yourself becoming more irritable or anxious over small things, snapping at loved ones or feeling overwhelmed by the simplest of tasks. Poor sleep does not just affect your energy; it also takes a toll on your emotional stability. Over time, this can deepen into feelings of depression or heightened stress, where everything seems harder to handle than it should be.

Your body sends signals too. You may notice catching colds more frequently or taking longer to recover from minor illnesses. That is because poor sleep weakens your immune system, making you more vulnerable to infections. At the same time, your body's response time slows down, leaving you feeling clumsy or less coordinated.

The physically effects of poor sleep are hard to ignore. You might find yourself gaining weight no matter how well you are eating or exercising. This happens because sleep influences the hormones that control hunger, often leading to cravings for sugary or high-calorie foods. In addition, there is that revealing sign we all recognize—dark circles or puffy eyes, which are visible markers of restless nights.

If you are waking up multiple times during the night, struggling to stay asleep, or tossing and turning, those are red flags too.

Frequent waking prevents your body from entering the deep, restorative stages of sleep, leaving you exhausted no matter how long you stay in bed.

The impact of poor sleep extends to relationships and physical well-being. You might notice a decrease in libido owing to the fact that your body is prioritizing survival over anything else. If you consistently find yourself reaching for stimulants like coffee or energy drinks just to keep going, that is another sign your body is not getting the rest it needs.

Over time, this dependence on caffeine only makes the problem worse, perpetuating a cycle of sleeplessness and daytime fatigue.

As the issue deepens, you may find yourself forgetting things more often—where you left your keys, important deadlines, or summaries of meetings. Sleep is essential for memory consolidation, so when you are not getting enough, your brain cannot properly store information. This mental decline becomes more noticeable over time, affecting both your personal and professional life.

All of these signs, from mood swings to forgetfulness to constant fatigue, are your body's way of telling you that something is not right. If you listen closely, you will notice that poor sleep does not just happen at night; it spills over into every waking moment, affecting your health, emotions, and your ability to function. By paying attention to these signals, you can start to take steps to restore your sleep quality and, with it, your overall well-being.

WHAT CAUSES THE CONDITION OF INSOMNIA?

Insomnia as a sleep disorder manifests through a range of symptoms that affect both sleep and daytime functioning. Its impact can be subtle or severe, gradually wearing down an individual's physical and mental health.

Experts do not fully understand why insomnia occurs, but the current understanding is that this condition involves an interplay of many factors. Some of these factors may be direct causes, while others could simply contribute to its development.

The symptoms of insomnia can vary but often include daytime fatigue, irritability, and difficulty concentrating, all of which further underscore the importance of addressing this condition.

Sleep scientists classify insomnia based on two key factors:
The Duration factor and **Nature-of-Cause factor**

1. Duration

a. **Acute Insomnia:** This is short-term and often lasts for a few days to weeks. It is usually temporary and may resolve on its own or with lifestyle adjustments.
b. **Chronic Insomnia:** This is long-term, persists for at least three months or longer, and can significantly affect quality of life.

1. Nature of the Cause

a. **Primary Insomnia:** This occurs on its own, with no underlying health issue contributing to the sleep disturbances.
b. **Secondary Insomnia:** Occurs as a symptom of another condition, such as stress, depression, or medical issues.

1
THE DURATION FACTORS:
Acute or Chronic Insomnia

Insomnia symptoms, whether acute or chronic, generally fall into the following categories:

a. **Difficulty Sleeping:** Trouble falling asleep, staying asleep, or waking up too early.

a. **Daytime Effects:** Lingering exhaustion, lack of focus, irritability, or impaired functioning during the day.

a. **Long-Term Sleep Disruption:** Persistent sleepless nights that affect long-term health and quality of life.

(a)
DIFFICULTY SLEEPING
(Duration factor)

When you struggle to sleep, that is a key symptom of insomnia. There are three main ways this happens with people commonly shifting between them over time:

1. Initial (sleep onset) insomnia:

This means you have trouble falling asleep.

One of the most common symptoms of insomnia is the struggle to fall asleep. As night falls, your mind may race with thoughts, worries or incapable of relaxing. The body might feel tired, yet sleep remains elusive. There may be difficulty falling asleep or a restless start to sleep. This restlessness can lead to:

- **Long Delays in Sleep Onset:** It can take 30 minutes or more to fall asleep, leading to frustration and anxiety about not getting enough rest.
- **Increased Alertness at Night:** Instead of winding down, the mind may become more active as the night progresses, making it even harder to drift off.

1. *Middle (maintenance) insomnia:*

This form causes you to wake up in the middle of the night but allows you to fall back to sleep. It is the most common form, affecting almost two-thirds of people with insomnia.

For those with frequent awakenings or interrupted sleep, staying asleep can be as challenging as falling asleep. Throughout the night, they may experience:

- **Multiple Awakenings:** Insomniacs often wake up several times during the night, sometimes for no apparent reason. These interruptions can be brief or last long enough to make it difficult to return to sleep.
- **Difficulty Returning to Sleep:** After waking up, individuals may lie awake for extended periods, unable to regain the peaceful slumber they need.

1. *Late insomnia (early waking):*

This form indicates that you wake up too early in the morning and cannot fall back asleep. You wake up earlier than necessary, often before the body has had sufficient rest. This early rising is not refreshing and leaves the individual:

- **Feeling Unrested:** Despite waking up early, the individual

may feel groggy, tired and dissatisfied with the amount of sleep they have received.
- **Unable to Fall Back Asleep:** Even if they have the opportunity to sleep longer, they find it impossible to return to sleep once they have awakened.

(b)
Daytime effects
(Duration factor)

Insomnia is much more than just struggling to fall asleep at night. Its impact reaches deep into the waking hours, leaving a trail of exhaustion that affects every aspect of life. The lingering effects of sleepless nights become painfully clear during the day, manifesting in a variety of ways that interfere with both mental and physical well-being. These effects extend beyond the night into the day and manifest through cognitive effects, mood disturbances, physical symptoms, impact on performance, coping mechanisms, and social withdrawal.

Since you need sleep to perform at your best, these disturbances commonly lead to symptoms that affect you while awake.

One of the most noticeable effects is the cognitive fog that clouds the mind. Concentration becomes a constant battle, as simple tasks at work, school, or home suddenly feel overwhelming. Insomniacs often find themselves struggling to focus, with their productivity plummeting. It affects memory, making it difficult to recall important details, stay organized, or manage day-to-day responsibilities. The mental sluggishness caused by insomnia can create a sense of frustration, as the simplest of activities require extra effort.

Beyond the mental toll, mood disturbances take hold. Even minor annoyances can ignite irritability, making it hard to interact with others. Social relationships may start to suffer, as insomniacs find themselves snapping at friends, family, or co-workers over trivial issues.

Nevertheless, it does not end there. Chronic insomnia can also lead to deeper emotional struggles, such as depression or anxiety. The constant exhaustion may fuel feelings of sadness or hopelessness, while the inability to rest properly can cause persistent worry and unease.

The body, too, pays the price for sleepless nights. Physical symptoms often include relentless headaches, with tension building up over time. Digestive issues may emerge as well—bloating, nausea, and a loss of appetite become common complaints. Insomnia also heightens sensitivity to pain, making even the smallest discomforts feel unbearable. Over time, the physical toll of insomnia adds another layer of stress to the daily experience, leaving individuals feeling worn out and fragile.

The consequences of insomnia are often glaring in professional or academic settings. Decreased performance becomes inevitable, with fatigue leading to a noticeable drop in productivity. Deadlines become harder to meet, and mistakes more frequent—some of which may have serious consequences. For those dealing with chronic insomnia, the workplace or school can become a place of dread, as the struggle to keep up with daily demands feels like an uphill battle.

In an effort to cope, many insomniacs turn to behavioural adaptations that can sometimes backfire. Excessive napping during the day might seem like a quick fix, but it often disrupts the natural sleep-wake cycle even further, making it harder to fall asleep at night. Others may start relying on sleep aids or alcohol to help them drift off, but this can lead to dependency, making the situation worse in the end.

As insomnia drags on, it can also lead to social withdrawal. Fatigue, irritability, and a lack of energy often cause people to retreat from social gatherings or avoid activities they once enjoyed. Relationships with friends, family, and co-workers may begin to fray as mood swings, forgetfulness, and emotional distance take their toll.

Over time, insomnia can isolate individuals, making it harder to maintain the social connections that are so vital to emotional health.

In short, insomnia is a pervasive condition that reaches far beyond the nighttime hours. Its effects ripple through every part of life, creating a cycle of physical, mental, and emotional exhaustion. The challenges insomniacs face don't simply end when the sun rises; they carry forward into every waking moment, making it clear that sleep isn't just a luxury—it's a necessity for overall well-being.

(c)
Long-Term Sleep Disruption (Duration factor)

The characteristics of insomnia symptoms are also significant. If your symptoms exhibit certain traits, you may be experiencing chronic insomnia. The characteristics include:

Circumstances: A diagnosis of chronic insomnia requires the presence of insomnia without factors that would disrupt your ability to sleep (such as changes in work schedule, life events, etc.). Diagnosing chronic insomnia demands experiencing sleep difficulties despite having adequate time and a suitable environment to sleep.

Frequency: Chronic insomnia entails experiencing insomnia frequently, at least three times per week.

Duration: Chronic insomnia persists for a minimum of three months.

Explanation: The insomnia is not occurring due to substances or medications (including both medical and nonmedical drugs) or other sleep disorders. Other medical or mental health conditions also cannot entirely account for your inability to sleep.

2
THE NATURE-OF-CAUSE FACTORS

This refers to any causal factor that remains constant over time. One cause contributes to the emergence of another cause through certain influences. The nature-of-cause factors refer to the underlying roots that contribute to a particular result or situation. These factors can be intricate, multifaceted and interrelated, often involving a blend of biological, environmental, psychological and social influences.

Biological Factors

Biological causes arise from the body's physiological processes, including genetics, brain chemistry and hormonal changes. For example, genetic predispositions can affect the likelihood of developing certain conditions like anxiety. Hormonal imbalances or disruptions in the body's natural rhythms can also be significant biological contributors.

From a biological perspective, several key mechanisms contribute to the development of insomnia and they include:

- **Family history (genetics):**

Genetic predispositions can also influence the likelihood of developing insomnia. Studies have shown that insomnia tends to run in families, which suggests genetic influence. Certain genes involved in the regulation of neurotransmitters and sleep-wake cycles may increase susceptibility to insomnia. However, genetics alone is rarely the sole cause; environmental factors often interact with genetic predispositions to trigger the condition.

- **Brain activity differences:**

Individuals with insomnia may have brains that are more active or brain chemistry variations that affect their ability to sleep. This heightened brain activity can result in racing thoughts, heightened anxiety, or the inability to "shut off" mentally, making it difficult for individuals to fall asleep.

- **Medical conditions and Substance use:**

Certain medical conditions can cause or exacerbate insomnia. Chronic pain, restless leg syndrome, asthma, and gastrointestinal disorders like acid reflux can disturb sleep. Certain medications, including stimulants, antidepressants, and corticosteroids, can interfere with sleep and lead to insomnia. Additionally, substances such as caffeine, nicotine, and alcohol can affect sleep architecture and the ability to fall asleep or stay asleep. Caffeine for instance blocks adenosine receptors, which normally promote sleepiness. Alcohol may initially induce sleep but disrupts sleep later in the night, causing awakenings and poor sleep quality

Psychological Factors

Psychological causes involve the mental and emotional state of an individual. Stress, anxiety, depression and other mental health issues can significantly influence behaviours and outcomes. Cognitive patterns such as negative thinking or unrealistic expectations can also play a role.

The constant pressure from work, relationships, finances, or health concerns elevates stress hormones, keeping the brain in a state of heightened alertness that makes relaxation and sleep nearly impossible.

For individuals prone to racing thoughts or rumination, the mind can become a whirlwind of worries, regrets, or unresolved issues, making it nearly impossible to switch of when it is time to rest. This constant mental activity feeds into a cycle of insomnia, as the more a person struggles to fall asleep, the more anxiety they feel about not being able to sleep, which only worsens the condition.

Negative sleep associations, often built over time, can also be a major hurdle. After repeated experiences of sleepless nights, a person may begin to associate bedtime with frustration and anxiety, further cementing the insomnia cycle.

Social Factors

Social causes are rooted in an individual's interactions with others and society. These include relationships, cultural norms, socioeconomic status and support systems. Social isolation or pressure to conform to societal expectations can lead to significant stress, thereby affecting both the quality and quantity of sleep.

Social isolation is in relation with a range of health problems, including anxiety and depression, which can adversely affect sleep. Feelings of loneliness can lead to an abnormal state of increased responsiveness to stimuli and repetitive thinking or dwelling on negative feelings, making it harder for individuals to relax and fall asleep.

Engaging with others is essential for emotional regulation. Those who are socially isolated may lack opportunities for positive interactions, leading to increased feelings of stress and anxiety.

Societal expectations around performance, productivity, and success can create significant pressure, as individuals may feel compelled to meet high standards in their professional and personal lives, leading to stress and anxiety that disrupts sleep.

The fear of not meeting societal expectations can exacerbate feelings of inadequacy. This anxiety can result in racing thoughts at bedtime, preventing individuals from achieving a state of relaxation conducive to sleep.

In cultures where long working hours are the norm, individuals may struggle to find a balance between work and personal life. This imbalance can lead to chronic stress and insufficient downtime, negatively affecting sleep.

Environmental Factors

Environmental factors encompass the external conditions or stimuli that influence an individual's sleep quality and quantity. This includes physical surroundings such as noise, light, or temperature, as well as lifestyle factors like diet, exercise and exposure to toxins. Environmental stressors, such as a demanding job or an unstable living situation, can also contribute to various outcomes.

Life changes, whether positive or negative, can trigger insomnia by disrupting routines, altering emotional states, and introducing new stressors. Major life transitions, such as moving to a new city, starting a new job, or entering a relationship, can throw off established sleep patterns. The excitement or anxiety associated with these changes often keeps the mind active, thereby preventing the relaxation needed for sleep.

Similarly, difficult life events like the loss of a loved one, divorce, or financial problems can lead to profound emotional distress. Grief, sadness, or feelings of uncertainty can overwhelm the mind, making it hard to quiet racing thoughts at night. During such periods, emotional turmoil consumes the body and brain, making sleep elusive.

Additionally, lifestyle shifts, such as a change in work schedule, caregiving responsibilities, or having a baby, can cause a disruption in sleep habits. Night shifts, long hours, or the demands of caring for a newborn can lead to irregular sleep patterns, making it difficult for the body to maintain a healthy sleep-wake cycle. Over time, this misalignment can contribute to insomnia.

Even positive life events, like the excitement of a wedding, pregnancy, or a long-awaited vacation, can cause temporary insomnia. The anticipation, planning, and emotional highs of such events can keep the mind overstimulated, making it hard to unwind and fall asleep.

Often, these factors do not act in isolation but are interconnected (interconnectedness of factors). For example, environmental stress can exacerbate psychological issues or biological predispositions may interact with social factors to increase the likelihood of insomnia.

Understanding the nature-of-cause factors requires a holistic approach when considering how these various elements interact and contribute to the overall outcome. This understanding is crucial for effective prevention, diagnosis and treatment.

RISK FACTORS AND COMPLICATIONS

RISK FACTORS
What makes sleeplessness more likely?

Sleep disorders, often regarded as a mere inconveniences, can be deeply rooted in various risk factors. They may lead to a cascade of complications that affect nearly every aspect of a person's life. They can affect anyone, but certain risk factors heighten the likelihood of developing any sleep disorder. These factors encompass physical, psychological, and lifestyle elements, often interacting in complex ways to disrupt sleep.

Continuous stress from work, relationships, or financial worries can keep the mind in a heightened state of alertness, making it challenging to unwind at night. This persistent pressure creates a cycle where the body cannot fully relax, even during periods of rest.

Individuals with anxiety disorders are particularly susceptible to insomnia, as their minds become overwhelmed with persistent worries, intrusive thoughts, and excessive concerns. These mental disturbances can hinder relaxation, making it hard to fall asleep or stay asleep throughout the night, often resulting in chronic sleep deprivation and heightened anxiety symptoms.

Depression can disrupt sleep patterns, leading to either insomnia or excessive sleep. In cases of insomnia, feelings of sadness, hopelessness, and rumination can interfere with both falling asleep and staying asleep.

This creates a vicious cycle where the lack of rest exacerbates depressive symptoms, further intensifying emotional exhaustion and complicating daily life. Conversely, some individuals may sleep excessively as a means of escape.

As people age, they naturally experience shifts in their sleep patterns, including earlier bedtimes, waking up earlier and having lighter, more fragmented sleep. These changes can diminish the overall quality and duration of rest, making older adults more vulnerable to insomnia. Additionally, age-related health issues, medications, and decreased physical activity can further disrupt sleep, complicating their ability to achieve restorative rest at night.

Hormonal changes during menopause, particularly hot flashes and night sweats, can significantly disrupt sleep patterns, leading to insomnia. These sudden temperature fluctuations and discomfort at night often result in frequent awakenings, making it a challenge for menopausal women to attain uninterrupted, restful sleep, further affecting their overall health and well-being.

Shift work, frequent travel across time zones and inconsistent sleep-wake patterns can significantly disrupt the body's natural circadian rhythm, leading to insomnia. When the internal clock is thrown off balance, it becomes challenging to fall asleep or stay asleep at appropriate times, resulting in poor sleep quality, fatigue and long-term negative effects on overall health.

Habits such as excessive caffeine or alcohol consumption, heavy meals before bedtime, or exposure to unsafe and uncomfortable sleep environments can greatly interfere with the ability to fall asleep and stay asleep. These behaviours disrupt the body's natural relaxation process, making it harder to achieve restorative rest.

Drugs used to treat conditions like Attention-Deficit/Hyperactivity Disorder (ADHD), certain antidepressants and some asthma medications can have stimulating effects that hinder the ability to fall asleep.

These medications can increase alertness or cause restlessness, disrupting the body's natural capacity to wind down. Consequently, individuals may experience difficulty falling asleep or staying asleep, leading to fatigue and decreased overall sleep quality over time.

Certain over-the-counter medications, such as decongestants and some pain relievers, contain ingredients that can interfere with sleep. These substances may elevate heart rate, cause restlessness or disrupt the body's natural sleep cycle, making it harder to fall asleep or maintain restful, uninterrupted sleep throughout the night.

Living in noisy environments or areas with excessive night-light exposure can significantly disrupt sleep patterns, leading to insomnia. Constant noise can hinder deep, restorative sleep, while exposure to artificial light interferes with the body's natural circadian rhythm. Over time, these environmental factors make it challenging to fall asleep and stay asleep, negatively impacting overall sleep quality.

An uncomfortable mattress, unsuitable pillows or a bedroom that is too hot, cold or cluttered can hinder relaxation and make it difficult to fall asleep. These physical discomforts disrupt the body's ability to settle into a restful state, complicating the achievement of quality sleep and contributing to ongoing sleep difficulties.

COMPLICATIONS
The Far-Reaching Consequences of Insomnia

The far-reaching consequences of insomnia extend well beyond just feeling tired. As such, what may start as few sleepless nights can spiral into a range of physical, emotional, and cognitive challenges, affecting nearly every aspect of an individual's life. As insomnia persists, its effects ripple through daily routines, making once-simple tasks seem overwhelming and eroding both mental and physical well-being.

On the surface, insomnia can lead to fatigue, irritability, and difficulty concentrating. However, its long-term impact is much deeper. It increases the risk of chronic health conditions like heart disease, diabetes, and weakened immunity. Emotionally, insomnia intensifies stress, anxiety, and depression, trapping individuals in a cycle where the fear of not sleeping worsens the problem. Social relationships and work performance can also suffer, as sleeplessness makes it harder to focus, communicate, and handle everyday responsibilities.

A persistent lack of sleep can result in overwhelming tiredness during the day, making it challenging to remain awake, focused and alert. This ongoing exhaustion affects daily activities, leaving individuals feeling drained and unmotivated, which can lead to irritability or emotional instability.

Fatigue significantly hinders cognitive functions such as attention, concentration and memory. This decline in mental acuity results in decreased productivity at work or school, with tasks taking longer to complete and a higher likelihood of errors. Fatigue also raises the risk of accidents, whether in the workplace, while driving or during other critical activities.

The emotional toll of insomnia can slowly escalate, creating a cycle of frustration, anxiety, and even hopelessness. At first, the exhaustion from sleepless nights might just leave someone feeling irritable or on edge. However, as insomnia persists, the emotional strain begins to deepen, affecting not only how a person feels but also how they handle daily life.

A lack of sleep can intensify negative emotions, making it harder to regulate mood. Small inconveniences that once seemed manageable may suddenly feel overwhelming, leading to outbursts of anger or bouts of sadness. Over time, this emotional volatility can leave someone feeling like losing control of their own responses, which adds to their stress. Insomnia also disrupts the brain's ability to process and manage stress, which can amplify feelings of anxiety.

For many, the nightly battle with sleep becomes a source of dread. The anxiety of not knowing whether they will get enough rest creates a mental barrier, making it even harder to fall asleep. This constant worry can evolve into more serious emotional complications as feelings of isolation and helplessness grow. Left unchecked, the escalating emotional toll of insomnia can significantly reduce quality of life, affecting mental health as deeply as it does physical well-being.

The long-term damage insomnia can inflict on physical health is profound and far-reaching. Chronic sleep deprivation does not just leave a person feeling exhausted—it slowly wears down the body's systems, increasing vulnerability to a range of serious health problems. Over time, the lack of restorative sleep starts to affect the heart, immune system, metabolism, and overall well-being.

One of the most significant risks is the increased chance of developing cardiovascular diseases. Insomnia puts constant strain on the body by elevating blood pressure and increasing inflammation, both of which are key contributors to heart disease, stroke, and heart attacks. The longer someone goes without proper sleep, the higher his or her risk becomes.

Insomnia also disrupts the body's hormonal balance, particularly those hormones responsible for regulating hunger and metabolism. This imbalance can lead to weight gain and a heightened risk of obesity, which in turn increases the likelihood of developing type 2 diabetes. With a weakened metabolism and insulin resistance, managing blood sugar becomes increasingly difficult.

Furthermore, the immune system suffers from ongoing sleep deprivation. Without enough sleep to repair and regenerate cells, the body's defences weaken, making it harder to fend off illnesses. Over time, the repeated strain of sleep disorders significantly weaken physical health, leaving lasting damage if left untreated.

Insomnia, with its relentless grip on sleep, can significantly increase the risk of accidents, both at home and in the workplace. When someone is sleep-deprived, their reaction times slow, attention wavers, and decision-making becomes impaired. Even simple tasks can feel overwhelming, and the margin for error grows dangerously thin.

For instance, driving while sleep-deprived is one of the most hazardous outcomes of insomnia. Studies have shown that being awake for 18 to 24 hours can impair driving ability as much as being over the legal alcohol limit. Those suffering from chronic insomnia are more prone to drifting off shortly behind the wheel, leading to car accidents. The risks are not limited to the road; they also extend to workplaces, especially in environments that require focus and precision, like construction sites or factories.

Fatigue from insomnia can lead to mishandling equipment, missing crucial safety cues, or making costly mistakes that endanger not only the individual but also those around them.

Even at home, small tasks like cooking or climbing stairs can become risky when exhaustion lowers concentration. Insomnia's toll on physical and mental alertness turns everyday activities into potential dangers, emphasizing the importance of addressing the sleep disorder before accidents occur.

The effects of insomnia stretch far beyond the individual, often having a significant impact on relationships and social interactions. When sleepless nights become a regular occurrence, the resulting fatigue, irritability, and mood swings can take a toll on one's ability to connect with others.

A person struggling with insomnia may find themselves feeling more short-tempered or emotionally reactive, causing tension in relationships with family, friends, or co-workers. Simple conversations can easily escalate into misunderstandings, as the lack of sleep affects patience and emotional regulation. Over time, this emotional instability may create distance in close relationships, as loved ones struggle to understand the cause of these mood shifts.

Sleep deprivation also diminishes one's capacity to focus, making it harder to stay engaged in conversations or follow through on commitments. This can lead to feelings of isolation, as the individual withdraws socially, either due to exhaustion or due to frustration.

In the workplace, insomnia can weaken teamwork, as reduced cognitive function and attention to detail make it harder to collaborate effectively. Insomnia's long-term interpersonal impact can affect nearly every aspect of life, highlighting the need for proper management and treatment to maintain healthy, positive relationships.

The long-term cognitive effects of insomnia can gradually erode the sharpness of the mind, affecting everything from memory to decision-making. As sleepless nights accumulate, the brain struggles to function at its full capacity. Concentration becomes elusive, and tasks that once felt simple may now seem overwhelming. It is as if a mental fog settles in, clouding your ability to focus and process information clearly.

One of the most troubling cognitive effects is memory impairment. Without sufficient sleep, the brain cannot properly consolidate memories, making it harder to retain and recall information. Over time, this can affect both short-term and long-term memory, leaving you feeling forgetful and scattered.

Insomnia also hinders your ability to solve problems and make decisions. The lack of sleep diminishes your cognitive flexibility, meaning you are less able to adapt to new situations or think critically. Even simple decisions can feel like complex puzzles, further contributing to feelings of frustration.

Beyond these effects, prolonged insomnia can weaken emotional regulation. Irritability, mood swings, and heightened stress responses are common, making it harder to manage relationships or handle everyday challenges. Over time, the cognitive toll of insomnia can deeply affect both your personal and professional life, blurring the line between exhaustion and mental clarity.

Insomnia is far more than just a night problem. It is a condition with wide-ranging implications for both physical and mental health. The risk factors that contribute to insomnia are diverse and interconnected, thus making it essential to identify and address them early.

MANAGEMENT AND TREATMENT DIAGNOSIS

The diagnosis of your sleep disorder is a meticulous process that involves evaluating your sleep patterns, medical history, and overall lifestyle. It goes beyond merely recognizing sleepless nights and requires a comprehensive examination of various factors to identify the underlying causes. The process typically starts with an in-depth consultation, during which your healthcare provider will ask about the duration and severity of your sleep disorders, possible triggers, and how it affects daily functioning. The healthcare provider will review your medical history to assess any conditions, such as anxiety, depression, or chronic pain that might contribute to the problem.

Physical examinations and laboratory tests may follow to rule out medical conditions like thyroid disorders or iron deficiencies that can disrupt sleep. In some cases, you may be required keep a sleep diary to track sleep habits, while the doctor might recommend a sleep study to monitor your brain activity and diagnose disorders like sleep apnea. This thorough process helps determine the most effective treatment approach for you.

The treatment approaches include but not limited to the following:

1. **Initial Assessment**
2. **Physical Examination**
3. **Sleep Studies**
4. **Sleep Questionnaires**
5. **Differential Diagnosis**

Initial Assessment: The First Step towards Understanding the Root Cause of your sleeplessness

The journey to diagnosing insomnia often begins with an in-depth discussion between the insomniac and healthcare provider. This initial assessment is vital in identifying the nature of the sleep difficulties and the factors contributing to them.

The provider will inquire about the patient's sleep habits, including how long it takes to fall asleep, how often they wake up during the night and how early they rise in the morning. They will also ask about the quality of sleep, how refreshed the patient feels upon waking up, in addition to the impacts on daytime functioning.

Patients typically maintain a sleep diary for one to two weeks. In this diary, they log when they go to bed, when they wake up, the number of times they awaken during the night and any daytime naps. This record offers valuable insights into sleep patterns and helps identify any triggers or patterns associated with insomnia.

The healthcare provider will review the patient's medical history to identify any conditions that might contribute to insomnia, such as chronic pain, asthma or other medical issues. They will also inquire about any medications the patient is taking, as some drugs can disrupt sleep.

Given that mental health significantly influences sleep, the healthcare provider will assess for conditions like depression, anxiety and stress, which are common contributors to insomnia. They might ask about recent life changes, emotional well-being and any stressors that could be affecting sleep.

Physical Examination: Ruling out Other Causes of your sleeplessness

A physical examination is often one of the first steps in treating insomnia, as it helps rule out any underlying health issues that may be causing sleep difficulties. During this process, your healthcare provider will check your vital signs, such as heart rate, blood pressure, and overall physical health. They will be on the lookout for conditions like heart disease, respiratory problems, or hormonal imbalances, all of which can interfere with sleep.

If something seems off, your doctor may suggest additional laboratory tests to dig deeper. For instance, they might check for an iron deficiency, which can sometimes lead to restless leg syndrome, a condition that causes discomfort in the legs and often disrupts sleep. In addition, doctors may request other blood tests to identify potential imbalances, deficiencies, or medical conditions that contribute to sleeplessness.

This thorough examination is crucial in determining whether your insomnia is because of a larger health issue. By addressing these underlying causes, your healthcare provider can create a more effective treatment plan that not only targets the insomnia but also improves your overall health, setting you on the path to a better, more restful sleep.

Sleep Studies: A Deeper Dive into your Sleep Patterns

If the initial assessment shows that insomnia stems from an underlying sleep disorder, the healthcare provider will recommend conducting a sleep study, commonly referred to as polysomnography.

A sleep lab usually performs this test, monitoring the patient's sleep overnight. Body sensors track brain waves, heart rate, breathing patterns, oxygen levels and body movements during sleep. This study helps identify conditions like sleep apnea, restless leg syndrome or periodic limb movement disorder, which can disrupt sleep.

In some cases, doctors conduct a simple sleep study at home, especially if they suspect sleep apnea. The patient uses portable equipment to monitor breathing patterns, oxygen levels and heart rate while sleeping in their own bed.

Sleep Questionnaires: Quantifying your Sleep Problems

Several standardized questionnaires can assist in evaluating the severity of insomnia and its impact on daily life. These tools offer a more structured approach to assess sleep quality and the extent of sleep disturbances.

Insomnia Severity Index (ISI) questionnaire evaluates the nature, severity and impact of insomnia. It includes questions regarding difficulties in falling asleep, staying asleep, waking up too early and the extent to which sleep issues affect daily functioning and quality of life.

Epworth Sleepiness Scale gauges daytime sleepiness, which can indicate how much insomnia is influencing a person's ability to remain awake and alert during the day.

Pittsburgh Sleep Quality Index (PSQI) evaluates sleep quality over a one-month period, examining aspects such as sleep duration, sleep efficiency and the presence of sleep disturbances.

Differential Diagnosis:

Identifying the Root Cause of your sleeplessness

One of the most challenging aspects of diagnosing insomnia is differentiating it from other sleep disorders or conditions with similar symptoms. The healthcare provider will consider other potential diagnoses and will work to determine whether insomnia is primary (occurring independently) or secondary (resulting from another condition).

Sleep Apnea is characterized by pauses in breathing during sleep, which can lead to frequent awakenings and poor sleep quality. A sleep study is often required to confirm this diagnosis.

Restless Leg Syndrome (RLS) is a condition that induces an uncontrollable urge to move the legs, often resulting in sleep disturbances. Symptoms typically worsen at night and can delay sleep onset.

Depression and Anxiety are mental health conditions that closely link with insomnia. A comprehensive psychological assessment helps ascertain whether insomnia is a symptom of an underlying mental health disorder.

Substance Use Disorders like the consumption of alcohol, caffeine, nicotine or any illicit drugs can lead to sleep issues. The healthcare provider will evaluate substance use that might be contributing to insomnia.

TREATMENT

The treatment of insomnia is a journey towards reclaiming restful nights and restoring balance in daily life. It involves a combination of strategies tailored to your individual needs, addressing both the underlying causes and the symptoms of sleeplessness. The goal is not only to help you fall asleep but also to create lasting improvements in your sleep quality and overall well-being.

Once all the detailed information about your sleep disorder is gathered, your healthcare provider will diagnose the type and severity of insomnia and develop a personalized treatment plan.

Primary Insomnia: Your insomnia is primary if does not link to another medical or psychological condition. Treatment will focus on cognitive behavioural therapy for insomnia (CBT-I), sleep hygiene education, and possibly short-term use of sleep aids.

Secondary Insomnia: If insomnia is secondary to another condition such as sleep apnea, chronic pain or depression, treatment will focus on addressing the underlying condition in addition to improving sleep.

Chronic vs. Acute Insomnia: The duration and frequency of insomnia symptoms will determine whether the diagnosis is chronic (lasting more than three months) or acute (short-term). Chronic insomnia often requires more comprehensive treatment strategies.

Some causes of insomnia are preventable, while others may occur due to obscure reasons. There are various ways to treat sleep disorders,, ranging from simple lifestyle changes and habits to different medications.

The main approaches to treating sleep disorders are:

1. **COGNITIVE BEHAVIOURAL THERAPY**
2. **LIFESTYLE AND HOME REMEDIES**
3. **ENVIRONMENTAL ADJUSTMENTS**
4. **ADDRESSING UNDERLYING MENTAL HEALTH CONDITIONS**
5. **MEDICATIONS**
6. **PROFESSIONAL SUPPORT**
7. **ALTERNATIVE AND COMPLEMENTARY THERAPIES**

1
Cognitive Behavioural Therapy

Cognitive Behavioural Therapy is an evidence-based treatment that assists individuals in addressing the thoughts and behaviours that contribute to sleep issues. It can help you modify unhelpful or unhealthy ways of thinking, feeling and behaving. It employs practical self-help strategies that can immediately enhance your quality of life.

Key Components of Behavioural Therapy for Insomnia include:

- **Cognitive Restructuring:**

This component of CBT-I aids individuals in identifying and challenging negative thoughts about sleep, such as "I will never be able to fall asleep" or "I cannot function without eight hours of sleep." By reframing these thoughts into more positive and realistic ones, it alleviates the anxiety surrounding sleep, making it easier to relax and fall asleep.

- **Sleep Restriction:**

This type of therapy limits the time spent in bed to the actual amount of time you sleep. This helps consolidate sleep and enhance sleep efficiency. By creating mild sleep deprivation, it strengthens the body's natural sleep drive, ultimately leading to longer and restorative sleep.

- **Stimulus Control Therapy:**

This approach aims to associate the bed with sleep rather than wakefulness. It encourages you to link your bed and bedroom with sleep and not with activities like watching TV or working. Individuals should to go to bed only when sleepy, to get out of bed if they cannot sleep within 20 minutes, and to reserve the bed for sleep and intimacy only, avoiding reading, watching TV or worrying.

- **Relaxation Techniques:**

This teaches relaxation methods such as deep breathing, progressive muscle relaxation, or guided imagery to help reduce anxiety and stress that may interfere with sleep. It calms the mind and body before bedtime. Reducing physical tension and quieting the mind makes it easier to transition into sleep.

- **Sleep Hygiene Education:**

This provides guidelines for creating a sleep-friendly environment and establishing a regular sleep routine, such as maintaining a consistent sleep schedule and avoiding stimulants like caffeine and nicotine close to bedtime.

- **Biofeedback:**

This employs monitoring devices to help you gain awareness and control over physiological functions such as heart rate and muscle tension.

Cognitive Behavioural Therapy is highly effective for treating chronic insomnia, often yielding long-lasting results. It does not rely on medications, thereby reducing the risk of side effects or dependency.

It also adapts to different sleep needs and preferences in line with your specific sleep issues. This therapy focuses on changing the thoughts and behaviours that contribute to sleeplessness.

Insomniacs can seek Cognitive Behavioural Therapy through a Healthcare Provider Referral, Online Programs and Apps, In-Person Therapy and Self-Help Materials.

Lifestyle and Home Remedies

Certain lifestyle changes and home remedies can be effective in managing sleep disorders.

Go to bed and wake up at the same time every day even on weekends. This helps regulate your body's internal clock. Engage in calming activities before bed such as reading, taking a warm bath or practicing relaxation techniques. Avoid stimulating activities, screens or heavy meals close to bedtime.

Make your bedroom comfortable. Keep it cool, quiet and dark. Invest in a good mattress and pillows that support a restful night's sleep. Avoid bright screens (phones, computers, TV) at least an hour before bed. Consider using blue light filters or glasses at night. Exposure to natural light during the day can help regulate your sleep-wake cycle.

Limit caffeine and nicotine intake, especially in the afternoon and evening. Avoid heavy or large meals, alcohol and sugary snacks close to bedtime. Engage in activities that signal your body it is time to wind down like listening to calming recitations or practicing gentle stretches.

Engage in regular physical activity, but try to avoid vigorous exercise close to bedtime. Even light activities like walking or yoga can improve sleep quality. Practice relaxation techniques such as deep breathing, meditation, progressive muscle relaxation or mindfulness. Consider journaling to clear your mind before bed.

If you take naps, keep them short (20-30 minutes) and avoid napping late in the afternoon. Try to get sunlight exposure and stay active throughout the day to help regulate your sleep cycle.

These lifestyle and home remedy strategies can often help improve sleep quality and reduce the impact of insomnia on your daily life. It may take some time to see significant improvements, so be patient and consistent with your efforts.

3
Environmental Adjustments

Environmental adjustments can play a crucial role in treating various sleep disorders by creating sleep-friendly environments that can significantly enhance the quality of your sleep.

Ensure your mattress and pillows are comfortable and supportive. Replace them if they are old or uncomfortable. Use soft, comfortable and breathable bedding that keeps you at a pleasant temperature throughout the night.

Use blackout curtains or shades to keep your room dark. Consider using an eye mask if necessary. Dim the lights in your home as bedtime approaches to signal to your body that it is time to wind down. Avoid screens (phones, computers, TVs) at least an hour before bed or use blue light filters or night mode settings.

Use a white noise machine, fan or a smartphone app to mask disruptive sounds. If you are sensitive to noise, consider using earplugs. Keep your bedroom cool within the ideal temperature range considered optimal for sleep. Ensure good airflow and ventilation in the room.

Keep your bedroom clean and free from dust and allergens. Consider using an air purifier to improve air quality if you have allergies or sensitivities. Consider using essential oils such as lavender, chamomile or sandalwood for their relaxing properties. Use a diffuser or spray a small amount on your pillow.

Keep your bedroom tidy and free of clutter to foster a peaceful environment. Ensure your bedroom feels secure and safe. If needed, implement additional locks or security measures to enhance your sense of comfort.

Use the bed solely for sleep and intimacy, avoiding activities such as watching TV, eating or working in bed. Establish a consistent routine to signal your body that it is time to sleep. This could involve activities like taking a warm bath, reading a book or practicing relaxation exercises.

By making these environmental adjustments, you can create a more conducive setting for restful sleep and effectively manage insomnia.

4
Addressing Underlying Mental Health Conditions

Mental healthcare plays a crucial role in treating sleep disorders, particularly when linked to stress, anxiety, depression or other mental health conditions.

Relaxation techniques such as deep breathing, progressive muscle relaxation, guided imagery and mindfulness meditation can alleviate stress and anxiety.

Mindfulness-Based Stress Reduction is a structured program that teaches mindfulness meditation to help manage stress and anxiety, thereby enhancing sleep.

Try this guided imagery drill:

Find a comfortable position, whether sitting or lying down, in a quiet space where you will not be disturbed. Gently close your eyes and take a moment to settle in. Now, bring your attention to your breathing. Take a deep breath in through your nose, allowing your abdomen to expand fully. Hold for a moment, and then exhale slowly through your mouth. With each breath, feel yourself becoming more relaxed, letting go of any tension.

Imagine a place that brings you peace and happiness. It could be a sun-drenched beach, a serene forest, or a cosy room. Picture this scene as vividly as you can. What colours do you see? What sounds fill the air? What scents linger around you?

Engage your senses further. If you find yourself at the beach, feel the warmth of the sun on your skin and hear the gentle rhythm of the waves. Breathe in the salty sea air, letting it refresh you.

Allow yourself to explore this tranquil environment. Walk along the shoreline, feel the soft sand beneath your feet, or find a shaded spot under a tree to relax. Take your time in this moment, savouring the peace surrounding you.

As you immerse yourself in this scene, notice any thoughts or worries that arise. If your mind starts to drift, gently guide it back to your peaceful place, focusing on the calm and serenity around you.

After a few minutes of exploration, begin to prepare to return. Start to bring your awareness back to the present. Wiggle your fingers and toes, and take a deep, grounding breath. Slowly open your eyes when you are ready.

Take a moment to notice how you feel after this experience. Carry this sense of calm with you as you continue your day, knowing that you can return to this peaceful place whenever you need to.

Learning to prioritize tasks and managing time effectively can greatly alleviate stress. Developing strategies to address challenges, such as setting achievable goals, breaking tasks into smaller steps, and practicing mindfulness, can also help reduce stressors in life. Cultivating these skills enhances resilience and overall well-being.

In today's fast-paced world, mastering the art of prioritizing tasks, managing time effectively, setting achievable goals, and breaking tasks into smaller steps can significantly boost productivity.

To start with prioritizing tasks, consider using the Eisenhower Matrix. Imagine categorizing your tasks into four quadrants: in the first, you find the urgent and important tasks that demand immediate attention. In the second, there are important but not urgent tasks, which you can schedule for later. The third quadrant contains urgent but not important tasks that you should delegate if possible, while the last quadrant holds tasks that are neither urgent nor important and which you can eliminate.

Another helpful technique is the ABC Method. Here, you assign an "A" to high-priority tasks, "B" to medium, and "C" to low-priority ones. This way, you can focus on completing the most critical tasks first.

When it comes to managing your time effectively, try time blocking. Picture your day divided into specific time slots dedicated to particular tasks. This structured approach helps you maintain focus and minimizes the temptation to multitask. You might also find the Pomodoro Technique beneficial—working for 25 minutes followed by a 5-minute break, and after four cycles, taking a longer break. This method can enhance your concentration and prevent burnout.

Limit distractions as much as possible. Identify what tends to pull your attention away, whether it is notifications or a noisy environment, and create strategies to minimize these interruptions.

Setting achievable goals is equally important. Utilize the SMART framework to ensure your goals are Specific, Measurable, Achievable, Relevant, and Time-bound. This clarity keeps you focused and accountable. Consider creating a vision board or using an app to visualize your progress, as this can serve as motivation.

Breaking tasks into smaller steps is crucial for making them more manageable. Think of chunking: take larger projects and divide them into smaller, actionable steps. For example, instead of simply stating, "write a report," break it down into tasks like "outline sections," "conduct research," and "write the introduction."

Each day, identify two to three key tasks you want to accomplish. This focused approach helps maintain momentum. Finally, at the end of each week, take a moment to review what you have accomplished. Reflect on what worked and what did not, and adjust your strategy as needed.

By integrating these techniques into your routine, you will enhance your ability to prioritize tasks, manage your time wisely, set realistic goals, and break down projects into manageable steps, ultimately leading to greater productivity and fulfilment.

Joining groups for individuals with insomnia or related mental health issues can offer support and shared experiences. Attend one-on-one sessions with a therapist to address specific concerns and to create personalized strategies in a treatment plan.

Joining support groups and seeking counselling can be transformative steps on your journey toward healing and personal growth.

Support groups offer a safe and welcoming space for individuals facing similar challenges, whether related to mental health, grief, addiction, or life transitions. In these groups, members share their experiences, providing mutual support and learning valuable coping strategies from one another. This sense of community helps reduce feelings of isolation, fosters understanding, and cultivates hope.

Counselling, in contrast, provides a more structured environment where you can explore your thoughts and feelings with a trained professional. A counsellor can help you identify underlying issues, develop coping mechanisms, and set personal goals. In therapy sessions, you will have the opportunity for deep reflection, gaining insights into your behaviours and emotions.

Both support groups and counselling offer significant benefits. They create connections with others who understand your experiences, fostering a sense of belonging. Engaging in these settings can empower you to take charge of your healing journey.

Moreover, you will learn practical skills for managing stress, improving communication, and enhancing emotional resilience. Sharing your experiences in a supportive environment validates your feelings and helps you realize that you are not alone.

Together, support groups and counselling form a comprehensive network of support, promoting resilience and facilitating your personal growth.

Understanding the vital connection between sleep and mental health can significantly inspire individuals to enhance their sleep hygiene and overall well-being. By recognizing how sleep influences emotional and psychological states, individuals are empowered to adopt effective strategies and habits that improve both sleep quality and mental health, resulting in a healthier lifestyle.

5
Medications

Various types of medications can assist you in falling or staying asleep. While Cognitive Behavioural Therapy for Insomnia is the preferred long-term solution, medications may be appropriate for short-term relief, especially when immediate improvement is required.

Many sleep medications are for short-term use due to the risks of dependence and side effects. Consider addressing the underlying causes of insomnia, such as stress, anxiety or poor sleep habits, in addition to using medications. Always consult a healthcare provider before starting any medication to ensure it is suitable for your situation and to discuss potential risks and benefits.

Regular follow-ups with a healthcare provider are essential to monitor the medication's effectiveness and make any necessary adjustments.

Be aware of potential interactions with other medications or health conditions. Provide your healthcare provider with a complete list of all medications and supplements you are taking.

While medications can be beneficial, combining them with non-medication strategies such as Cognitive Behavioural Therapy for Insomnia (CBT-I), good sleep hygiene and lifestyle modifications often leads to the best outcomes for managing insomnia.

6
Alternative and Complementary Therapies

Relaxation technique such as yoga, combined with mindfulness and meditation, can help promote relaxation and improve sleep quality. They foster a deeper connection between mind and body by enhancing self-awareness. Incorporating yoga into your daily routine, even just a few times a week, can lead to significant improvements in physical health, mental clarity and emotional well-being.

In the hustle and bustle of modern life, finding moments of peace can often feel like a daunting challenge. However, incorporating relaxation techniques into your daily routine can help you cultivate a sense of calm and well-being. Here are several methods that can serve as pathways to tranquillity, each offering its unique benefits.

Deep Breathing is one of the simplest yet most effective ways to relax. Picture yourself in a quiet space, free from distractions. Begin by taking a deep breath in through your nose, allowing your abdomen to expand fully. Hold that breath for a few seconds, feeling the fullness of air within you. Then, exhale slowly through your mouth, releasing tension with each breath out. Repeat this process, focusing solely on your breathing. With each inhalation, imagine drawing in peace and calm; with each exhalation, visualize letting go of stress and anxiety. This technique not only calms the mind but also reduces physical tension.

Next, consider Progressive Muscle Relaxation. This technique is particularly beneficial if you carry tension in your body. Find a comfortable position, either sitting or lying down. Start with your toes—tense the muscles as tightly as you can for a few seconds, then release. Feel the difference between tension and relaxation. Gradually work your way up your body, tensing and then relaxing each muscle group—your feet, legs, abdomen, arms, and finally your face. This method helps you become more aware of where you hold tension and teaches your body how to let go.

Meditation is another powerful tool for relaxation. Set aside a few minutes each day to sit in a quiet space. Close your eyes and focus on your breath, noticing the rhythm of inhaling and exhaling. If your mind begins to wander, gently guide your attention back to your breath or a calming mantra. Over time, this practice can help you develop a greater sense of inner peace and clarity, allowing you to approach life's challenges with a more relaxed mindset. Guided meditation apps like Headspace or Calm can provide helpful structure if you are new to the practice.

Another effective method is Mindfulness, which encourages you to stay present in the moment. Take a moment to observe your surroundings. Notice the colours, sounds, and sensations. Try practicing this anywhere—while eating, walking, or even during a conversation. By focusing on the here and now, you can reduce feelings of anxiety and stress, thereby creating a sense of groundedness.

Incorporating Yoga into your routine can also promote relaxation. This ancient practice combines movement, breath, and meditation. Try gentle stretches and poses that encourage relaxation. As you move through the poses, focus on your breath and let go of any lingering tension in your body. Even a short yoga session can significantly improve your mood and state of mind.

Visualization is a technique that taps into the power of your imagination. Find a quiet spot and close your eyes. Picture a peaceful scene—perhaps a serene beach, a lush forest, or a tranquil mountain landscape. Engage all your senses: imagine the sound of waves, the scent of pine trees, or the warmth of the sun. Allow yourself to immerse fully in this imagery, letting it wash over you. This mental escape can provide profound relaxation and rejuvenation.

Finally, consider Walking in Nature. Taking a stroll outdoors not only benefits your physical health but also nurtures your mental well-being. Pay attention to the sights and sounds around you—the rustling leaves, the chirping birds, the feeling of the ground beneath your feet. This connection to nature can ground you and create a deep sense of relaxation.

Incorporating these relaxation techniques into your life can help you find balance and peace amid the chaos. Experiment with different methods to discover which ones resonate most with you, and allow yourself the gift of relaxation. As you create space for calm in your life, you may find that you can navigate challenges with greater ease and resilience.

Many herbs and supplements can aid in treating insomnia. Certain herbs, such as valerian root, chamomile and lavender promote relaxation and sleep. While many of these are common and well known, it is best not to assume that an herb or supplement is automatically safe for you. You should consult a healthcare provider about herbs and supplements before taking them. This helps you avoid possible side effects or interactions, especially if you have any medical conditions or take other medications.

It is also important to remember that while medications can assist with sleep, they may negatively affect your sleep cycle. Sleep quality, not just quantity, is crucial. This means you should use medications, even over-the-counter ones cautiously.

For centuries, people have turned to herbs and supplements as natural remedies for sleeplessness, seeking alternatives to pharmaceuticals. One of the most renowned options is valerian root, known for its ability to enhance sleep quality and shorten the time it takes to fall asleep. This herb works by increasing levels of gamma-aminobutyric acid, or GABA, in the brain, promoting a sense of calm.

Chamomile is another popular choice, often enjoyed as a soothing tea. Its mild sedative effects can help ease anxiety and create a sense of relaxation, making it easier to drift off to sleep.

Then there is lavender, frequently used in aromatherapy. The scent of lavender improves sleep quality and increase deep sleep, making it a favourite for those seeking a peaceful night.

Melatonin, a hormone that regulates our sleep-wake cycles, is also a common supplement for those struggling with insomnia, particularly beneficial for those dealing with jet lag or circadian rhythm issues.

While not an herb, magnesium is essential for good sleep. It helps regulate neurotransmitters, and researchers have linked low levels to sleep disturbances, making it a key nutrient for those seeking better rest.

However, it is important to approach these remedies with caution. Consulting a healthcare professional is essential, as dosages and potential interactions with medications vary. Additionally, addressing lifestyle factors like sleep hygiene, diet, and stress management is crucial for achieving restful sleep.

Ultimately, while herbs and supplements can offer significant benefits for sleeplessness, they work best as part of a holistic approach that includes thoughtful lifestyle adjustments and possibly other therapeutic interventions.

Whether through cognitive behavioural therapy, medications or complementary therapies, the goal is to restore a healthy sleep pattern and enhance overall quality of life. With the right combination of treatments and ongoing support, individuals with insomnia can find relief and reclaim the restorative sleep they need to thrive.

THE PRACTICAL OUTLOOK TO SLEEPLESSNESS

What to expect if you have sleep disorders

Sleeplessness is typically not a major concern. Most individuals who experience sleep disorders may feel tired or not quite their best the following day, but that feeling often improves once they obtain sufficient quality sleep over time. They may feel sleepy, fatigued or low on energy during the day, struggling with concentration, memory and decision-making.

Chronic insomnia is disruptive. While it is usually not dangerous, it can still negatively affect your life in numerous ways. If you have insomnia, the experience can feel like an exhausting battle against your own mind and body where sleep seems just out of reach. This struggle affects not only your nights but also your days by casting a shadow over your energy, mood and overall well-being.

If you find yourself lying awake at night, staring at the clock as the minutes turn to hours, you might be stepping into the world of insomnia. At first, it might just seem like a restless night with tossing and turning, trying to find a comfortable position, or calming your racing thoughts. Nevertheless, as the nights go on and sleep continues to evade you, you start to feel the weight of insomnia settling in.

During the day, you might find it hard to concentrate, your thoughts cloudy, and your patience shorter than usual. Small tasks may feel overwhelming, and the lack of energy starts to creep into everything you do. Even if you manage to sleep for a few hours, it rarely feels refreshing.

As the sleepless nights add up, your mind feels the strain also. Worries about not being able to sleep begins to build up, making you dread bedtime, and turning it into a source of anxiety rather than relief.

You may try to force sleep, but the harder you try, the more elusive it becomes.

Sleep disorders can be unpredictable in their duration, ranging from a brief encounter to a prolonged struggle. For some, theymay last only a few nights, triggered by stress, a major life change, or even excitement. This can be a form of acute insomnia—a short-term disruption that typically resolves on its own once the underlying cause passes. It is frustrating but temporarily feels like a storm that eventually clears.

However, when sleeplessness lingers for weeks, months, or even longer, it transitions into chronic insomnia. This type of insomnia is more complex and deeper issues such as ongoing stress, underlying medical conditions, or long-standing habits that interfere with sleep is often tied to it. In chronic cases, sleep becomes a nightly challenge, where no amount of exhaustion guarantees rest, and the struggle feels never-ending.

The length of time insomnia can last will depend on its root cause. For some, adjusting lifestyle habits, addressing health concerns, or reducing stress can help restore a healthy sleep pattern. However, for others, insomnia may last longer, demanding more structured treatment and attention.

Whether it is fleeting or persistent, insomnia's impact can be profound and will keep affecting your daily life until there is proper management of the underlying issues.

The Lingering Shadow of Stress and Anxiety

Stress and anxiety significantly influence the duration of insomnia by creating a complex interplay that affects both mental and physical health. When you experience stress, your body enters into a state of heightened arousal. Hormones like cortisol and adrenaline flood your system, preparing you for a "fight or flight" response to sudden life changes or looming deadlines. This physiological reaction can trigger a brief period of insomnia, making it difficult to relax and fall asleep.

As anxiety takes hold, racing thoughts and persistent worries can make it nearly impossible to quiet your mind at night. Whether you are preoccupied with work, relationships, or health concerns, these thoughts can keep you awake, prolonging the time it takes to fall asleep and leading to awakenings that are more frequent during the night.

Stress and anxiety also disrupt your sleep architecture. They affect the various stages of sleep, resulting in fragmented sleep and a decrease in restorative sleep stages like deep sleep and Rapid Eye Movement sleep.

This disruption leaves you feeling unrefreshed by exacerbating the feelings of fatigue and irritability.

Over time, you may develop a conditioned response to your bedroom. If insomnia becomes a recurring issue, you might begin to associate your bed with sleeplessness and worry. This conditioning turns your sleeping environment into a source of stress rather than a sanctuary for relaxation, further prolonging insomnia.

Negative cognitive patterns play a role as well. The drama of exaggerating the consequences of not sleeping sufficiently can perpetuate anxiety and stress, thereby creating a vicious cycle where worries about sleeplessness lead to even greater difficulty in falling asleep.

The impact of insomnia due to stress and anxiety extends into our daily lives. Concentration, mood, and overall functioning can be racked with pain as the increasing stress levels create a feedback loop that makes insomnia last longer. Physical symptoms, such as muscle tension, headaches, and gastrointestinal issues, can manifest because of stress and anxiety. These discomforts make it even harder to find rest and that adds another layer of complexity to our sleep struggles.

You may also find yourself avoiding situations that provoke stress or anxiety, such as social gatherings or work responsibilities. This avoidance can create additional stress and further limit your opportunities for relaxation.

When chronic stress and anxiety diminish your coping mechanisms, you might feel overwhelmed by daily challenges. In such cases, relaxing, even at night, can feel impossible. Poor sleep intensifies the feelings of stress and anxiety, while increased stress and anxiety worsen sleep difficulties. This cycle can make insomnia last much longer than it would otherwise.

The Hidden Contribution of Underlying Medical Conditions

Insomnia can be a persistent companion when underlying medical conditions are at play. Imagine someone struggling to fall asleep, not just for a few nights, but for weeks or even months. This is not just a passing phase of sleeplessness but also a chronic battle that stretches on because of deeper health issues beneath the surface.

For someone living with chronic pain, like arthritis (inflammation of one or more joints, causing pain and stiffness that can worsen with age), or fibromyalgia (widespread muscle pain and tenderness), every movement in bed becomes a reminder of the discomfort, making it hard to drift into sleep. The pain does not fade with nightfall but instead, it lingers, keeping the person awake and restless. Over time, this constant struggle to sleep becomes a long-term ordeal.

Then there are those whose minds refuse to quiet down. Anxiety, depression, or the lingering effects of trauma, can turn the night into a time of racing thoughts and heavy emotions. No matter how tired they are, their minds spin, replaying worries and fears, making it impossible to find rest. Night after night, this cycle repeats, stretching insomnia into something more enduring.

For others, it is a matter of their bodies working against them. Nervous system disorders such as Parkinson's or Alzheimer's disease can wreak havoc on the brain's natural sleep-wake cycle. What should be a simple process of falling asleep then becomes a constant struggle that turns peaceful nights into rare occurrences.

In addition, there are those whose hormones or respiratory systems will not cooperate. Sudden hot flashes or night sweats, for example, may awaken a woman going through menopause and disrupt her sleep just when she needs it most. On the other hand, someone with asthma or sleep apnea may find themselves jolted awake, gasping for air, unable to stay in a deep, restful sleep.

In all of these cases, the insomnia is not just about trouble sleeping; it is about an ongoing battle with an underlying condition. Individuals will find sleep elusive, and insomnia will continue to be a long-term part of life until they manage or treat those conditions.

The Influence of Environmental Factors

Environmental factors significantly influence the duration and severity of insomnia by creating an interplay between your surroundings and your ability to achieve restful sleep. Understanding how these elements affect your sleep can lead to meaningful changes that promote better rest.

Light exposure plays a crucial role in regulating your sleep-wake cycle. Natural light during the day helps your body's internal clock function properly by making it easier to fall asleep at night. However, insufficient natural light can disrupt this rhythm, leading to difficulties at bedtime. On the other hand, excessive exposure to artificial light, particularly the blue light emitted by screens, can hinder production of the sleep hormone vital for restorative sleep. This interference can cause problems falling asleep and result in shorter sleep duration.

Noise levels in your environment can also have a profound effect on your sleep quality. Persistent noise, whether from traffic, loud neighbours, or other sources, can interrupt your sleep and make it harder to stay asleep. Even low-level, persistent sounds can fragment your rest and reduce its overall quality. In contrast, a quieter environment promotes relaxation and deeper sleep, allowing you to rest more soundly. Utilizing white noise machines or earplugs can help mask disruptive sounds, thereby creating a more peaceful sleeping atmosphere.

Temperature is another essential factor. The temperature of your sleeping environment greatly affects your comfort. If your room is too hot or too cold, it can lead to discomfort, making it challenging to fall asleep or stay asleep throughout the night. Ideally, the temperature should be between 60 to 67 degrees Fahrenheit (15 to 19 degrees Celsius).

Additionally, the materials of your bedding and sleepwear contribute to your overall comfort and ability to regulate your body temperature while you sleep. Wearing comfortable, cosy sleepwear can create a sense of relaxation and readiness for sleep by serving as a part of bedtime ritual that mentally prepares you for rest. Soft textures and familiar garments can signal to your body that it is time to wind down.

The comfort of your sleep environment matters immensely as well. A supportive mattress and a comfortable pillow are fundamental to achieving restful sleep. An uncomfortable sleeping surface can lead to physical discomfort and frequent awakenings, which prolong insomnia. High-quality sheets and blankets that match your comfort preferences can further enhance your sleeping environment.

People often overlook air quality, even though it is a critical factor. Poor air quality or inadequate ventilation can lead to discomfort and difficulty sleeping. Ensuring good air circulation and using air purifiers can create a more conducive sleeping environment. Additionally, allergens like dust mites, mould, and pet dander can trigger allergies and respiratory issues, thereby making it difficult for you to sleep. Keeping your bedroom clean and free from allergens is essential for achieving better rest.

Maintaining a consistent sleep environment helps signal to your body that it is time for rest. However, changes in your sleep environment, such as traveling or sleeping in unfamiliar places, can disrupt your routine and intensify insomnia. Engaging in stimulating activities before bed, like intense exercise or stressful work, can further affect your ability to wind down and fall asleep. Establishing a calming pre-sleep routine can help counteract these effects.

Our social environment is another important aspect to consider. The behaviour and habits of those we live with can significantly affect our sleep. A snoring partner, children who wake up during the night or even loud conversations, can disrupt our ability to rest. Living in shared spaces or communal environments, such as dormitories, may introduce disturbances that affect our sleep quality.

A stressful work environment, whether due to demanding deadlines or a toxic atmosphere, can carry over into your home life and hinder your ability to unwind.

Devices like TVs, computers, and smartphones can disrupt your ability to fall asleep. Establishing technology-free zones in your bedroom can help create a more peaceful atmosphere conducive to rest.

Substance Use: The Double-Edged Sword

Substance abuse can turn insomnia into a relentless, long-term struggle. Picture someone relying on drugs or alcohol to cope with stress or to find an escape route, only to find that sleep keeps becoming harder and harder to reach.

Stimulants like amphetamines give an initial rush of energy, keeping the mind buzzing late into the night. At first, it might seem harmless or just a temporary high, but over time, the brain becomes unable to switch off. Even long after the drug wears off, sleep becomes elusive with restless nights stretching into weeks, or even months.

Alcohol, on the other hand, might seem like a shortcut to relaxation. After a few drinks, sleep may come easily, but it is deceptive. As the night wears on, the body struggles to stay in a deep, restorative sleep. Instead, the person wakes up frequently, feeling groggy and unrested. For someone who drinks regularly, this poor sleep pattern becomes a cycle that is hard to break, turning a few restless nights into chronic insomnia.

Then there are sedatives and sleeping pills, often taken in the hope of getting better sleep. At first, they might seem like the perfect solution, but the body soon starts to depend on them. As tolerance builds, the drugs become less effective, and the insomnia returns to an unusual extent. Worse yet, trying to stop these medications can bring on withdrawal symptoms including intense anxiety, restlessness, and of course, sleeplessness that lingers.

For those battling addiction, withdrawal from substances like opioids or benzodiazepines is particularly brutal. The brain, starved of the chemicals it has come to rely on, struggles to find its natural balance. Insomnia can last for weeks or months as the body slowly adjusts, stretching the road to recovery even further.

Even after the individual quits, the damage to their brain's sleep mechanisms can be long lasting. The delicate balance of neurotransmitters that regulate sleep has been altered, and it takes time, sometimes years, for the body to recover fully. In this way, substance abuse turns what could have been a brief struggle with insomnia into a prolonged battle, one that can linger even in sobriety.

The Vicious Cycle of Psychological Conditioning

Psychological conditioning can turn insomnia into a drawn-out, exhausting ordeal. Imagine someone lying awake night after night, staring at the ceiling, unable to sleep. It initially seems like just a bit of frustration, but over time, something more insidious like anxiety takes root.

Every night, as bedtime approaches, the negatively affected individuals begin to dread bedtime. Their mind start racing, anticipating another sleepless night and this anxiety grows stronger. Instead of looking forward to rest, they feel a sense of stress, their body tensing as they prepare for another battle with insomnia. The simple act of lying down becomes a trigger for worry, making it even harder to relax, let alone drift off to sleep.

As the nights go by, bad habits begin to form. Instead of using the bed as a place of rest, they start watching TV, scrolling through their phone, or even working in bed. The brain, once wired to associate the bed with sleep, now sees it as a place for activity and alertness. Therefore, when they finally try to sleep, the bed feels anything except restful. It is as if the body has forgotten how to shut down in that space.

For some, life's stresses only add fuel to the fire. The worries of the day carry over into the night, creating an abnormal state of increased responsiveness to stimuli that is marked by various physiological and psychological symptoms, where the mind and body are too alert to sleep. The original stress might fade, but the body has already learned to stay on high alert at bedtime, and the insomnia remains.

As they try to make up for lost sleep, they might start napping during the day or going to bed earlier than usual, desperate to catch up. Nevertheless, these efforts backfire, disrupting their natural sleep-wake cycle and reinforcing the insomnia even more.

Soon, the bedroom itself becomes a battleground. Just walking into the room or lying down sends a signal to the brain: "Stay awake". What used to be a space for peace and rest is now a place of tension, where the body fights sleep rather than welcome it.

This cycle of psychological conditioning traps the individual in a prolonged struggle with insomnia. It takes time and effort to break free, to retrain the brain, and rebuild the positive associations with sleep that have been lost. Only by addressing these deep-seated patterns can they finally begin to reclaim their nights and find rest once more.

The Path to Resolute Treatment and Intervention

The mode and timing of treatment interventions can significantly influence the duration of insomnia. Early intervention, particularly with effective treatments like Cognitive Behavioural Therapy for Insomnia (CBT-I), can lead to a quicker resolution of insomnia.

If insomnia remains untreated, it may develop into a chronic condition. The longer it lasts, the more entrenched the sleep difficulties can become, making them harder to address.

Conversely, seeking treatment early and identifying the right combination of therapies can help reduce the duration of insomnia. Whether through behavioural changes, therapy, or medication, timely intervention can disrupt the cycle of sleeplessness and restore healthy sleep patterns.

As indicated earlier, Cognitive Behavioural Therapy for Insomnia (CBT-I) is a structured approach that addresses the underlying thoughts and behaviours that contribute to insomnia. When initiated early, this therapy can help reshape a person's relationship with sleep, often leading to quicker and more lasting improvements. Its focus on sleep education and practical strategies empowers individuals to take control of their sleep patterns, often reducing insomnia duration significantly.

Medications may offer immediate relief from insomnia symptoms, but their effectiveness depends on how they are used. Short-term use can help individuals manage acute episodes, while long-term reliance without addressing underlying causes may lead to a cycle of dependency. If individuals pair medications with behavioural therapies early on, they can transition away from pharmacological solutions more quickly, thereby reducing the overall duration of insomnia.

Implementing good **sleep hygiene practices** like establishing a regular sleep schedule and creating a relaxing bedtime routine can have a rapid impact on sleep quality. The introduction of these practices at the onset of difficulties can help prevent the escalation of insomnia.

Introducing Relaxation Techniques such as mindfulness or progressive muscle relaxation is effective, especially when integrated into a treatment plan early. By promoting relaxation, these techniques help reduce anxiety and stress, allowing for quicker improvements in sleep duration.

Addressing insomnia at its onset can prevent it from becoming chronic. If individuals seek help promptly, they can adopt effective strategies before the insomnia becomes entrenched.

Sticking to a treatment plan consistently over time amplifies its effectiveness. For instance, if you apply sleep hygiene practices regularly from the start, you can create a stable sleep environment that encourages quicker recovery. Regular follow-ups allow for adjustments to the treatment plan based on how the individual responds. This adaptability can lead to a faster resolution of symptoms, as you can fine-tune interventions for optimal effectiveness.

When considering the duration of interventions, it is important to differentiate between short-term and long-term approaches. While short-term interventions may provide quick fixes, they often fail to address the root causes of insomnia. On the other hand, long-term strategies, such as sustained cognitive behavioural therapy or lifestyle modifications, may require more time but can lead to significant and lasting improvements in sleep quality. This, in turn, reduces insomnia duration.

Continuous support and follow-up after initial interventions can reinforce new sleep habits and help prevent relapse. Regular check-ins or ongoing therapy provide accountability and motivation, sustaining the progress made in improving sleep.

Personalizing treatment plans based on individual needs can greatly enhance their effectiveness. Factors such as age, underlying health conditions, and specific sleep issues should count in when designing an intervention plan. Personalized approaches tend to be more successful in addressing insomnia and can lead to quicker resolution of symptoms.

Moreover, combining various interventions such as lifestyle changes, cognitive behavioural therapy and medication when necessary creates a comprehensive strategy that targets multiple facets of insomnia. This multifaceted approach often results in quicker and more effective resolution of sleep issues.

Engaging social support systems can also enhance the effectiveness of interventions. Involving family members or friends in the process provides additional support and accountability, making it easier to adhere to new sleep habits. This social reinforcement can lead to improved outcomes and a shorter duration of insomnia.

The effectiveness of interventions has close ties to individual readiness to change. Those who are motivated and willing to engage with the intervention are likely to see quicker improvements in sleep. Encouraging individuals to track their sleep patterns, mood, and lifestyle factors can increase awareness and promote adherence to intervention strategies.

COPING MECHANISMS

Coping with stress and life's challenges is something we all face, but the ways we choose to handle these pressures can make all the difference. Some coping mechanisms are healthy because, they provide a positive way to manage difficult emotions whiles others are unhealthy for the reason that they offer only temporary relief that often leads imprudence in the end, owing to the fact that we fail to consider the possible results of our actions.

For many, exercise and physical activity is a vital coping mechanism for sleeplessness. Whether it is a brisk walk, a calming yoga session, or an intense workout. Physical movement helps release endorphins, which are the body's natural mood enhancers that can alleviate pain, lower stress, improve mood, and enhance our sense of well-being. Regular physical exercises not only reduce stress but also improve sleep, boost energy, and offer a mental respite from daily challenges, in ways that can improve our sense of control, coping capability and self-esteem.

In the same way, mindfulness and meditation provide a powerful way to regain control over a racing mind. Taking time to focus on breathing, or simply being present in the moment, can help reduce anxiety and stress. These techniques train the mind to tune out distractions and negative thoughts in order to foster a sense of calm and balance.

Another key to coping well with sleeplessness is leaning on social support. Whether it is talking with a close friend, confiding in a family member, or seeking out a professional counsellor, sharing the load with someone you trust can make challenges feel less overwhelming.

Having someone to listen or offer perspective is often the initial relief needed to move forward.

Healthy hobbies also offer an escape from stress. Whether it is painting, gardening, reading, volunteering, or engaging in club activities that bring joy, can be incredibly therapeutic. These creative outlets provide a break from life's stresses while giving a sense of accomplishment and fulfilment.

For those who thrive on structure, time management becomes essential. By organizing tasks, setting clear priorities, and breaking down big projects into smaller and manageable steps, it is easier to maintain control over an industrious life. Proper time management reduces the feeling of being overwhelmed and helps avoid unnecessary stress.

Some people find solace in journaling or putting their thoughts and feelings down on paper as a way to break down emotions. Writing out frustrations, anxieties, or even positive experiences can help clarify thoughts and relieve emotional pressure. It is a healthy release and a personal space for reflection.

Others turn to positive self-talk as a way of conditioning the mind to replace negative, self-defeating thoughts, with constructive and encouraging words. Reminding yourself that you can handle challenges, and that setbacks are a normal part of life, helps build resilience and reduces the shady feelings of helplessness.

Equally important is the ability to set boundaries. Learning when to say "no", whether in personal relationships or at work, is key to protecting emotional and physical health. By maintaining limits, individuals can avoid burnout and preserve the balance needed for long-term well-being.

Unfortunately, not all coping mechanisms are beneficial. Some people turn to substance use, such as relying on alcohol, hard drugs, or smoking as a way to numb the stress. In their own class, these drugs produce a state of feeling intense happiness, excitement, or sense of well-being while relieving fear, tension, and anxiety. While these may offer a temporary escape, they often lead to addiction or worsen mental and physical health, thereby creating a vicious cycle of dependency and despair.

Others might develop unhealthy eating habits—overeating or undereating—as a way to handle emotional strain. While these eating behaviours provide comfort for a brief moment, they can lead to significant health issues and exacerbate stress over time.

One of the most common but damaging responses to stress is avoidance or withdrawal. Instead of facing problems head-on, some choose to avoid them by isolating themselves or procrastinating. This provides short-term relief but often leads to deeper feelings of anxiety and frustration as unresolved issues pile up.

For some, oversleeping or sleep deprivation becomes a way to escape. Some may sleep excessively to avoid facing their problems, while others may be too anxious to sleep at all. Both extremes take a toll on health and can worsen stress.

In moments of high tension, some people lash out, resorting to aggression or irritability as a coping mechanism. While venting frustrations might feel like a release, it damages relationships and often escalates conflicts, which can lead to more stress in the end.

Finally, there are those who turn to compulsive behaviours like uncontrollable desire to shop, gamble, or engage in risky activities, in an attempt to cope with their emotions. These habits may provide temporary relief, but they often lead to greater problems, such as financial strain or feelings of guilt.

Ultimately, how we choose to cope determines whether we build resilience or create more problems for ourselves. Healthy coping mechanisms, such as exercise, mindfulness, social support, and setting boundaries, help us navigate life's challenges in a way that promotes mental, emotional, and physical well-being. On the other hand, unhealthy mechanisms, such as substance use, avoidance, or aggression, may offer quick relief but often lead to bigger issues down the road.

The mechanics of coping is a lifelong necessity, but the key is choosing methods that support long-term health and happiness, rather than those that simply mask the pain in the moment.

Living with insomnia can be challenging, but numerous strategies and resources can assist you in managing your condition and maintaining a good balance between sleep and wakefulness.

To improve your insomnia and overall sleep architecture, some of the most crucial actions you can take revolve around practicing good sleep hygiene.

Set and follow a sleep schedule

Imagine you are trying to improve your sleep. You know the key is to establish a routine that suits your body's needs. First, you think about how much sleep you truly need to feel rested. Seven to nine hours is the typical range for adults, but you tune into your own body's cues.

Once you figure that out, the next step is choosing a wake-up time that works for your schedule. Whether it is for work, school, or your morning routine, having a consistent wake-up time sets the foundation for your day. You make a commitment to wake up at the same time every day and even on weekends. It may sound tough, but soon enough, your internal clock will adjust.

Now, you do the math. Let us presume you need eight hours of sleep, and you want to wake up at 7:00 AM. You realize that your bedtime needs to be 11:00 PM. This bedtime becomes your goal, but it is not just about lying down at 11:00 PM and hoping for the best. You create a wind-down routine. You dim the lights, put away your phone, and maybe read a book or take a warm bath. The routine itself signals to your body that it is time to rest.

Your bedroom environment matters too. You make it as cosy as possible: cool, quiet, and dark. You can acquire blackout curtains, adjust your pillows, or even try out a white noise machine. It all adds up to creating the perfect sleep haven.

One thing you also need to realize is the impact of immediate bedtime activities on how well you sleep. Activities you directly engage in as bedtime approaches. Caffeine is a no-go in the evening, and you avoid late-night meals that leave you feeling uncomfortable. You have heard that exercise helps with sleep, so you start working out during the day, but you avoid doing it too late at night, since that might keep you wired and alert.

As tempting as it is to sleep in on weekends, you already know that consistency is key. You stick to your routine, waking up at the same time every day. Over time, your body adapts, and sleep comes more naturally. If you find yourself struggling at the initial stages of your sleep, try making gradual changes by moving your bedtime earlier by 15 or 30 minutes at a time until it feels right.

Finally, you learn to manage the stress that may keep you awake. You practice deep breathing, meditation, or mindfulness, whatever will help calm your mind before bed. With time and patience, you start to feel the benefits of a regular sleep schedule where you wake up feeling more refreshed, more energized, and ready to face each new day.

Give yourself time to wind down

Set aside the day's concerns before bedtime as much as you can. Allow for a buffer period between when you finish your day and when you go to bed. This can help you get into the right frame of mind for sleep.

As bedtime approaches, you start thinking about how to wind down and prepare for a restful night. You set a specific time, about 30 to 60 minutes before bed, to start your routine. It is a signal to your body that sleep is on the horizon.

You begin by dimming the lights around the house. This small change mimics the natural setting sun and gently encourages your body to produce melatonin, the hormone that helps you drift off to sleep. You make it a point to turn off your phone, computer, and television. The blue light from those screens, as you know, can mess with your brain's ability to unwind, so you decide to give yourself a break from them. Replace your phone with a traditional alarm clock to avoid the temptation of scrolling through social media or checking emails. Establish a rule to refrain from using your phone in bed or during the hour leading up to bedtime. Keep it out of reach by placing your phone across the room or in another room to reduce temptation.

With screens off, you pick up a book, maybe something light and calming. If reading feels too engaging, you opt for an audiobook, letting the soft voice of the narrator pull you into a relaxed state. Soon, you start to feel your mind slow down.

Next, you head to the bathroom for a warm shower or bath. The heat feels soothing, and as you step out into the cooler air, you notice your body naturally cooling down, and that is another signal that it is time to rest. This little shift in temperature helps make you drowsy.

You take a few moments to practice some deep breathing exercises, inhaling slowly through your nose and exhaling through your mouth. Alternatively, maybe tonight, you prefer some gentle yoga or light stretches to release any lingering tension in your muscles. As you breathe and stretch, you feel your body loosening up, and with each breathing out, you feel every stress from the day melt away.

A warm, caffeine-free beverage sounds nice, so you make yourself a cup of chamomile tea or warm milk. You take slow sips, savouring the warmth as it travels through your body, calming your mind further. If worries or tasks for tomorrow begin creeping into your thoughts, you grab a journal and jot them down. Once they are on paper, they no longer need to take up space in your mind.

To set the mood, you put on some soft, calming nature sounds in the background—maybe the sound of rain, ocean waves, or gentle wind through trees. The familiar rhythm lulls you closer to sleep and the noises from outside fade away.

As the final touch, you add a few drops of lavender essential oil to your pillow or turn on a diffuser. The soft, relaxing scent fills the air, adding another layer of peace to your bedtime ritual.

In the calm and quiet, you feel ready to fall asleep. By taking the time to unwind, you have allowed yourself to drift naturally into rest, leaving the day behind and preparing for tomorrow with a refreshed body and mind.

Get comfortable

Feeling comfortable is essential for achieving quality sleep. Adjust your sleeping environment, including lighting, sounds, and temperature. Ensure your bedroom is as comfortable as possible. Invest in a supportive mattress and pillow to provide proper support for your spine and avoid aches and pains.

Imagine settling into bed after all the aforementioned routines, your body sinking into a soft, supportive mattress, and with the perfect temperature surrounding you. As you adjust your pillow and stretch out, you feel your muscles begin to relax, tension melting away. In this moment of comfort, your body is telling you it is ready for sleep. You are not tossing or turning to find a better position, and the worries of the day fade as your mind begins to quiet.

As you drift off, your breathing slows and deepens, unrestricted by awkward angles or discomfort. Each intake of breath feels effortless. Your body, properly supported, stays still, and you do not wake up throughout the night from pressure points or lingering pain. Your sleep becomes peaceful and uninterrupted. The kind that lets your body truly rest and recover.

Medical Management

For some time, you've been struggling with restless nights, tossing and turning, unable to find the peace you need for a good night's sleep.

You have finally consulted with your doctor, who has provided a clear treatment plan customized for your needs. You begin to follow your prescription, perhaps, also engaging in alternative therapies designed to manage your symptoms.

As you stick to this plan, you start to notice changes. If you have been dealing with a sleep disorder, like insomnia, the treatments gradually help you fall asleep more easily and stay asleep longer. The medication balances your body's hormones, ensuring that melatonin and other sleep-regulating chemicals are in harmony as they guide you into restful sleep each night.

If chronic pain has been your issue, the treatments begin to ease that persistent discomfort, and like a shot, lying in bed is not a source of agony anymore. Your muscles loosen, your body relaxes, and sleep comes more naturally. The mental strain that often keeps you awake, including anxiety, depression, or stress, now becomes more manageable as you follow your therapy and medication routine.

Over time, the simple act of following your treatment plan creates a sense of consistency. You take your medications, follow your sleep schedule, and your body adjusts. There is no longer a struggle to get to sleep, as your body now knows what to expect. The recurrence of symptoms that used to wake you up in the middle of the night fades away, leaving you to experience undisturbed, restorative sleep.

By staying committed to your treatment, you realize how important it is for your overall well-being. Each night of quality sleep becomes a step toward better health, and in turn, your improved health supports even better sleep. It is a cycle, and all it took was **trust** and following that plan.

Emotional and Social Support

Picture this: after a long, exhausting day, you lie in bed, but sleep does not come easily. Your mind keeps racing, weighed down by worries and emotions you have kept bottled up. Then, you remember the conversations you have had with a close friend or family member and how they listened, understood, and helped ease the tension in your mind. Seeking that emotional support gave you a chance to release those pent-up feelings, making the load a little lighter.

With that weight off your shoulders, your stress starts to fade. Your mind, no longer overwhelmed, begins to calm down, and you feel a sense of security in the wake of knowing you are not alone in facing your challenges. This emotional stability allows your body to relax, and you slowly drift into sleep, free from the anxious thoughts that used to keep you awake.

Over time, your support network helps you cope with life's difficulties more healthily. Instead of staying awake at night, overthinking, or feeling isolated, you share your struggles. The connections you've built provide not just comfort but real solutions—whether it is a practical advice on better sleep habits or simply a reassuring word that helps you feel safe and secure.

That sense of belonging, of knowing you can lean on others, gives you emotional balance that helps you sleep more soundly. You are no longer lying in bed with feelings of loneliness or anxiety. Instead, you feel supported, which creates an environment where restful sleep is possible.

Each night, the emotional and social support you have sought becomes a vital part of your journey to quality sleep. With a calm mind, a secure heart, and the encouragement of those who care for you, sleep comes easier and with it, the energy to face the next day.

Education and Awareness

Let us be under the impression that your restless nights and constant fatigue is because of a specific sleep condition, insomnia to be precise. At first, it feels overwhelming, but as you begin to educate yourself, you realize that knowledge is your most powerful tool. The more you learn about your condition, the more empowered you feel to manage it.

You take it upon yourself to seek education and awareness about your health condition's symptoms, triggers and treatment options that will empower you to make informed decisions regarding your care. You then dive into consultation with your healthcare provider, engaging in research and soon, you have a tailored treatment plan designed just for you. Whether it is about adopting cognitive behavioural techniques for insomnia, you now understand what your body needs for sufficient sleep. With this information, you start to notice improvements—you sleep more soundly, and waking up no longer feels like a struggle.

Staying informed also helps you stay vigilant. You have learned the warning signs of worsening symptoms, and if your sleep starts to decline, you know when to adjust your treatment. This proactive approach allows you to catch issues early and prevent them from disrupting your rest.

The more you understand about your condition, the more committed you become to your own self-care. You stick to a sleep routine, make lifestyle changes, and avoid habits that interfere with your rest. Instead of feeling frustrated or anxious about your sleep problems, you feel calm and in control, knowing that you have the tools and knowledge to manage them.

You begin to feel more confident with each conversation that you have with your healthcare provider. You ask informed questions, understand your treatment options better, and make reliable choices that fit your needs. The clearer your communication, the more effective your treatment becomes.

Over time, this dedication to learning about your sleep condition not only improves your sleep but also safeguards your overall health. You are able avoid the long-term consequences of untreated sleep disorders, and each night of quality sleep sets you up for a healthier, more energized life.

When should I see my healthcare provider?

In addition to the physical benefits of regular doctor visits, there is also a psychological advantage to consider. Visiting the doctor can offer peace of mind, especially for those who are anxious about their health.

It can also enable the doctor to make accurate diagnoses and prescribe appropriate treatments.

Timely medical intervention can often prevent a minor issue from escalating into a major one. Knowing that you are taking steps to maintain your health can foster a sense of control and reduce worry.

Recognizing when to seek care is vital for preventing complications and sustaining a good health record.

Here are some situations under which you should consider seeking medical care:

> Persistent sleepiness during waking hours that is difficult to resist, **or**

> Brief episodes of falling asleep during waking hours (known as micro sleeps), particularly if they occur while working or driving, **or**

> Experiencing symptoms such as snoring, gasping, feeling breathless during sleep, leg discomfort, frequent urination at night, **or**

> If insomnia began after starting a new medication, **or**

> If over-the-counter medications are ineffective or you find yourself relying on them regularly, **or**

> If you have other conditions, including mental health issues or concerns that impact your sleep quality and duration.

When in doubt or uncertain about changes in your sleep pattern, or if you have symptoms that you do not understand, or you are concerned about, seek professional medical advice as soon as possible.

Your healthcare provider can help identify the underlying cause of your sleeplessness and suggest appropriate treatments or referrals to specialists if necessary.

What questions should I ask my doctor?

It is always better to err on the side of caution and seek care when uncertain. Your healthcare provider can offer guidance on whether your situation requires immediate attention or in a scheduled appointment.

You should consult your healthcare provider, especially, a primary care provider, if you notice that your sleep disorder has been lasting more than a few nights and/or if it begins to affect your daily routine, tasks and activities.

Consider asking the following questions to your healthcare provider when you observe abnormal changes in your sleep patterns.

> How do I tell if I am getting enough quality sleep?

> How are my current medications (if any) affecting my sleep?

> Is my physical health influencing my sleep and do I possibly have symptoms or another condition that is preventing me from getting enough rest?

> How can I determine if I have insomnia?

> What might be causing my insomnia?

> How can I manage my other health conditions alongside insomnia?

> What is the best treatment for me?

> How can I prevent insomnia?

It is essential to be honest and open about your symptoms, even if you feel embarrassed or shy. Clear and transparent communication between you and your physician or healthcare provider can help both of you make informed decisions about your health.

Sleep is something people often take for granted until they are not getting enough of it. Quality sleep is a critical component of your health. A lack of sufficient sleep can cause disruptions, both significant and minor, in your overall well-being. If you begin to experience any form of sleep disorder, consider speaking to your primary healthcare provider immediately.

Doctors can provide an accurate diagnosis based on your symptoms, medical history and diagnostic tests. This ensures that you fully understand what is wrong. Once diagnosed, they can prescribe the appropriate treatment, whether it involves medication, therapy or lifestyle changes. This targeted approach can help resolve the issue more effectively.

Early diagnosis and treatment can prevent ailments from worsening or leading to more severe health problems. Timely medical intervention can often stop a minor issue from escalating into a major one.

Doctors can offer expert advice on managing symptoms, preventing future issues and maintaining overall health. They can also provide information on lifestyle changes that may improve your condition.

Additionally, they can refer you to specialists, recommend further tests and provide information on support groups or other resources that might be beneficial.

Consulting a doctor can ease anxiety by providing clarity and reassurance regarding your health condition. Knowing that a professional is overseeing your care can be very comforting.

They can also customize their advice and treatment plans to your individual needs and circumstances by considering your medical history and any ongoing health issues.

Regular check-ups with a doctor allows for continuous monitoring of your condition, thereby ensuring that the treatment is effective and adjusting it if necessary.

Having a documented medical evaluation can be crucial for work, as it provides official evidence of your condition and treatment. Doctors can educate you about your ailment by helping you understand how it impacts your personal and professional life and what you can do to manage or alleviate symptoms.

Milton Keynes UK
Ingram Content Group UK Ltd.
UKHW030851111124
451035UK00001B/154